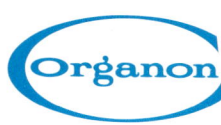

GW01558166

With Compliments

Organon Laboratories Ltd
Cambridge Science Park, Milton Road, Cambridge CB4 4FL
Tel: (0223) 423445

CHRONIC HYPERANDROGENIC ANOVULATION

CHRONIC HYPERANDROGENIC ANOVULATION

The Proceedings of the
First Organon Round Table Conference
Oss, 9–10 October, 1989

Edited by H.J.T. Coelingh Bennink
H.M. Vemer and P.A. van Keep

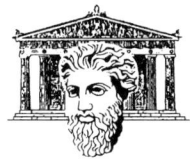

The Parthenon Publishing Group
International Publishers in Medicine, Science & Technology

Casterton Hall, Carnforth,
Lancs, LA6 2LA, UK

120 Mill Road, Park Ridge,
New Jersey 07656, USA

Published in the UK and Europe by
The Parthenon Publishing Group Ltd.
Casterton Hall
Carnforth, Lancs. LA6 2LA

Published in North America by
The Parthenon Publishing Group Inc.
120 Mill Road,
Park Ridge,
New Jersey, NJ, USA

Copyright © 1991 The Parthenon Publishing Group Ltd.

ISBN: 1-85070-322-1

Typeset by Lasertext Ltd., Stretford, Manchester
Printed and bound in Great Britain by
Butler & Tanner Ltd., Frome and London

Contents

List of principal participants and contributors

T. Bergh
Dept. of Obstetrics and Gynecology
Uppsala University
S-751 85 Uppsala
Sweden

M.H. Birkhäuser
Clinic of Obstetrics and Gynecology
Division of Gynecological Endocrinology
Universitäts-Frauenklinik
3012 Berne
Schanzeneckstrasse 1
Switzerland

M. Breckwoldt
Dept. of Obstetrics and Gynecology
Division of Clinical Endocrinology
University of Freiburg
Hugsterstrasse 55
D-7800 Freiburg im Breisgau
FRG

H.J.T. Coelingh Bennink
Organon International bv
Molenstraat 110
PO Box 20
5340 BH Oss
The Netherlands

A. Dunaif
Division of Endocrinology
Dept. of Medicine
Mount Sinai School of Medicine
One Gustave L. Levy Place
New York
New York 10029
USA

B.C.J.M. Fauser
Dept. of Obstetrics and Gynecology
Dijkzigt University Hospital
Dr. Molewaterplein 40
3015 GD Rotterdam
The Netherlands

M. Filicori
Center for Chronobiology of Reproduction
  and Reproductive Medicine Unit
University of Bologna
Italy

R. Fleming
Dept. of Obstetrics and Gynaecology
Queen Elizabeth II Building
Royal Infirmary
Glasgow G31 2ER
UK

S. Franks
Dept. of Obstetrics and Gynaecology
St. Mary's Hospital Medical School
London W2 1PG
UK

H.J. van Geldorp
Academisch Ziekenhuis Rotterdam
Dr. Molewaterplein 40
3015 GD Rotterdam
The Netherlands

K. Gordon
The Jones Institute for Reproductive
  Medicine
Dept. of Obstetrics and Gynecology
Eastern Virginia Medical School
855 West Brambleton Avenue
Suite B
Norfolk
Virginia 23510
USA

J.V.T.H. Hamerlynck
Dept. of Reproductive Endocrinology and
  Fertility
Academic Medical Center
Meibergdreef 9
1105 AZ Amsterdam
The Netherlands

M.J. Heineman
Dept. of Obstetrics and Gynecology
The Wever Hospital
6419 PC Heerlen
The Netherlands

F.M. Helmerhorst
Dept. of Obstetrics and Gynecology
University Hospital
Rijnsburgerweg 10
NL 2333 AA Leiden
The Netherlands

S.G. Hillier
Dept. of Obstetrics and Gynaecology
University of Edinburgh Centre for
  Reproductive Biology
37 Chalmers Street
Edinburgh EH3 9EW
UK

G.D. Hodgen
Academisch Ziekenhuis Rotterdam
Dr. Molewaterplein 40
3015 GD Rotterdam
The Netherlands

P.A. van Keep
Organon International bv
Molenstraat 110
PO Box 20
5340 BH Oss
The Netherlands

R.E. Lappöhn
Dept. of Obstetrics and Gynecology
Academisch Ziekenhuis Groningen
Oostersingel 59
9713 EZ Groningen
The Netherlands

T.J. McKenna
Dept. of Endocrinology and Diabetes
  Mellitus
St. Vincent's Hospital
Elm Park
Dublin 4
Ireland

M.I. New
Room N-236
Dept. of Pediatrics
The New York Hospital–Cornell Medical
  Center
525 East 68th Street
New York
New York 10021
USA

G. Schaison
Service d'Endocrinologie et des Maladies
  de la Reproduction
Hôpital Bicêtre
78 rue du Général Leclerc
94275 Le Kremlin Bicêtre
France

J. Schoemaker
Division of Reproductive Endocrinology
  and Fertility
Free University Hospital
De Boelelaan 1117
1081 HV Amsterdam
The Netherlands

R.W. Shaw
Academic Dept. of Obstetrics and
  Gynaecology
The Royal Free Hospital
Pond Street
London NW3 2QG
UK

H.M. Vemer
Organon International bv
Molenstraat 110
PO Box 20
5340 BH Oss
The Netherlands

M.A.H.M. Wiegerinck
Dept. of Obstetrics and Gynecology
Sint Joseph Hospital
5600 ML Eindhoven
The Netherlands

Preface

In 1989 Organon celebrated the 100th birthday of Dr Saal van Zwanenberg, the young industrialist who in 1923 founded the company. He did this in close cooperation with Professor Laqueur, the professor of pharmacology in Amsterdam.

Now, almost 70 years later, there is still considerable empathy between workers in Organon and those working in academia, an empathy which has in the past resulted frequently in joint efforts with shared successes and shared failures. In 1989 one of us (H.J.T. C.B.) took the initiative to organize a workshop conference on a subject that would be of interest to reproductive endocrinologists without being directly linked to Organon's present line of products. Thus, representatives from both worlds – the industry and academia – joined their knowledge, experience and creativity to explore the many aspects of the topic chosen for this conference, viz. chronic hyperandrogenism in women.

This volume contains the papers presented at the conference. Special thanks are due to Dr G. Hodgen who was an exemplary moderator in the final discussion session.

The Editors hope that these Proceedings, forming together a comprehensive survey of a complicated subject, will make interesting reading for the many pleasant contacts that Organon has all over the world, whether they are investigators, advisers, friends or prescribers of Organon's products. With the organization of this workshop conference and the distribution of this book, Organon wants to emphasize its commitment to that important field of medicine: Gynecology.

H.J.T. Coelingh Bennink
H.M. Vemer
P.A. van Keep

SECTION 1

Pathophysiology of chronic hyperandrogenic anovulation

1

Classification of chronic hyperandrogenic anovulation

B.C.J.M. Fauser

INTRODUCTION

In the original paper of Stein and Leventhal[1], the presence of bilaterally enlarged ovaries exhibiting multiple follicle cysts was described in seven women presenting with sterility, amenorrhea and masculinization. Ovarian wedge resection was considered to be the treatment of preference. This procedure also provided ovarian tissue, which enabled the diagnosis of Stein–Leventhal disease to be confirmed by microscopic examination. In the 1960s surgical procedures lost popularity, and it was reported that certain signs and symptoms of patients were frequently associated with polycystic ovaries at operation[2]. Consequently, more recently the diagnosis – referred to as polycystic ovary syndrome – was mainly based upon the presence of clinical symptoms, and ovarian abnormalities have been assumed. Chronic hyperandrogenic anovulation (CHA) represents the same clinical syndrome, emphasizing the presence of high androgen levels in combination with anovulation. Recently, pelvic ultrasonography has allowed non-invasive examination of ovaries on a large scale, which enables ovarian abnormalities in these patients to be re-examined[3].

At present CHA can be classified based on three main criteria: clinical presentation, biochemical characterization, and characterization of ovarian abnormalities (Table 1). Because in routine clinical practice diagnostic criteria should be simple and easy to implement, specific signs and symptoms together with hormone estimates in peripheral blood are considered to be of major importance. In this review, criteria which may be important for the diagnosis and classification of CHA are discussed.

CLINICAL PRESENTATION OF CHA

Most patients exhibiting CHA have a distinct clinical history with a normal menarcheal age, excessive hair growth and overweight before, and irregular menstrual cycles directly afer menarche[4]. Within families of patients with polycystic ovary syndrome there seems to be dominant transmission, with a

13

Table 1 Criteria for the classification of CHA

Clinical presentation
Patient history (initiation symptoms before/during puberty)
Family history
Signs and symptoms (infertility, hirsutism, obesity, anovulation)

Biochemical characterization
Peripheral blood;
   augmented LH/FSH ratios
   high androgen levels (T/SHBG ratio)
   hyperprolactinemia
   insulin resistance
Follicular fluid
Ovarian tissue/cell cultures

Characterization of ovarian abnormalities
Classical morphology
Laparoscopic inspection
Ultrasonography

---

variable type and degree of expression of symptoms, and hirsutism and oligomenorrhea as the main complaints[5]. In addition, hypertension, diabetes, insulin resistance and obesity occur more often in families of polycystic ovary syndrome patients, with endocrine abnormalities and disturbed testis function in male family members. Goldzieher and Axelrod[2] reviewed over 1000 patients described in literature with polycystic ovaries at operation, and calculated the incidence of infertility, hirsutism, amenorrhea and obesity to be 74, 69, 51 and 41%, respectively.

Overweight is considered to be an important clinical diagnostic criterion since it represents the capacity to convert androgens to estrogens in peripheral fat tissue. Weight is often expressed as BMI (body mass index; weight divided by height^2), and overweight is defined as BMI > 25. However, there is discussion as to what extent BMI adequately represents body fat content[6]. Skinfold thickness or underwater body weight may be more suitable for the accurate assessment of body composition. Hirsutism as a clinical sign of hyperandrogenemia, a main diagnostic criterion also, can be quantified according to criteria set by Ferriman and Gallway[7]. However, hair growth on some parts of the body may be dependent mainly on genetic factors, and therefore racial differences do occur. The above-mentioned discrepancy between clinical criteria and body fat content and hyperandrogenism may explain observed differences in the incidence of these signs in CHA.

BIOCHEMICAL CHARACTERIZATION OF CHA

Hyperandrogenemia is known to be involved in anovulation and the occurrence of polycystic ovaries in various clinical states such as congenital adrenal hyperplasia, androgen-producing tumors, Cushing's disease and long-term androgen treatment in female-to-male transsexuals. Controversy still exists, however, as to what extent androgen screening should be performed clinically for proper diagnosis of hyperandrogenism. Next to testosterone (T), assays of other steroids (such as androstenedione, dihydro-epiandrosterone, dihydrotestosterone, or 17-hydroxyprogesterone) could be performed. The determination of dihydroepiandrosterone sulfate (DHEAS) levels as an exclusive marker of adrenal androgen production is generally considered to be a useful addition, since it can distinguish between ovarian and adrenal androgen production, which may have important therapeutic consequences. Determination of sex hormone binding globulin (SHBG) allows calculation of the 'free androgen index' (T $\times$ 100/SHBG) which may adequately represent androgen activity[8].

Augmented luteinizing hormone/follicle stimulating hormone (LH/FSH) ratios have also been considered a key biochemical criterion for the diagnosis of polycystic ovary syndrome. Based on extensive work done by Yen and colleagues[9], we now know that this altered gonadotropin output mainly represents increased pituitary sensitivity due to altered steroid feedback. Absolute values for LH/FSH ratios, however, may depend on applied radioimmunoassays as well.

Hyperprolactinemia and insulin resistance can also be observed in a proportion of patients suffering from CHA. This will be discussed in subsequent chapters.

In the near future, further characterization of CHA syndromes may include hormone estimates in follicular fluid on a larger scale. These estimates may involve androstenedione/estradiol ratios as an index of granulosa cell function, estimates of radioimmunoactive and bioactive FSH levels as a indication of granulosa cell stimulation, and determination of various growth factors (such as insulin-like growth factor) as potential intraovarian regulators. Moreover, granulosa cell function could be characterized *in vitro* by culturing cells[10] or ovarian tissue.

CHARACTERIZATION OF OVARIAN ABNORMALITIES IN CHA

CHA diagnosis can be based upon the classical morphological criteria of Stein and Leventhal[1], exhibiting stroma hyperplasia, hyperthecosis, capsule thickening and cystic degeneration of follicles. At present, the availability of ovarian tissue for microscopy is rare, since surgical procedures are infre-quently performed. Moreover, a description of the distinct ovarian appearance of polycystic ovaries during laparoscopy is also rarely applied as a diagnostic procedure.

Ultrasonography represents a non-invasive technique to identify ovarian abnormalities in patients with polycystic ovary syndrome where diagnosis is based on clinical criteria (Table 2)[11-17]. Symmetrically enlarged cystic ovaries were found in 2.5% of a large group of patients presented for pelvic ultrasound[11]. In patients suffering from clinical symptoms of polycystic ovary syndrome, enlarged ovaries (one- or two-sided) were present in roughly 70%, and cystic structures could be observed within the ovaries in 30–70% (which may depend mainly on the quality of the ultrasound image) of cases. The reported maximum size of ovarian cysts was 10 mm, with a minimum

Table 2 Pelvic ultrasound in patients with polycystic ovary syndrome (PCOS)

| | | Ultrasound of ovary | | |
| | | | Ovarian cysts | |
Reference	Patients	Description	n	Size (mm)
Swanson et al.[11]	863 total	2.5% enlarged, cystic	6–16	2–6
Hann et al.[12]	28 PCOS	71% enlarged 39% cystic	—	< 10
Parisi et al.[13]	26 PCOS	70% enlarged, cystic	—	< 5
Orsini et al.[14]	50 PCOS	36% enlarged, cystic often same as normal	—	4–10
Adams et al.[15]	148 anovulation 25 hirsutism	56% polycystic (stroma ↑) 92% polycystic	> 10	2–8
Tabbakh et al.[16]	20 PCOS	70% enlarged 50% cystic	—	< 10
Yeh et al.[17]	104 PCOS	30% normal size 74% cystic	> 5	5–8

cyst number per ovary of five. In patients exhibiting polycystic ovaries by ultrasound (Table 3), oligo- or amenorrhea occurred in roughly 70%, and hirsutism in 50–60%. Although mean T and LH levels in the polycystic group are increased significantly[15], individual LH and T levels are above normal in only 40 and 22%, respectively[18].

CONCLUSIONS

It seems that chronic hyperandrogenic anovulation diagnosed on the basis of clinical criteria such as obesity, hirsutism, cycle abnormalities and hormone estimates in peripheral blood is a common expression of various underlying entities. Recent developments have allowed more accurate characterization

Table 3 Polycystic ovaries and clinical signs of polycystic ovary syndrome

Reference	Patients	Clinical findings
Adams et al.[15]	84	80% oligomenorrhea 50% hirsutism mean LH↑, mean T↑
Eden et al.[8]	68*	24% regular cycles 76% oligo-/amenorrhea
Conway et al.[18]	556	71% oligo-/amenorrhea 61% hirsutism 40% LH↑, 22% T↑

*Diagnosed by ultrasound and laparoscopy

of follicle maturation arrest by ultrasound, and of granulosa cell function by biochemical characterization of follicular fluid. These procedures may provide valuable additional information to further define ovarian abnormalities in polycystic ovary syndrome. This additional information may eventually enable the classification of ovarian hyperandrogenemia into subgroups, each with a distinct underlying defect. The classification of underlying abnormalities involved in anovulation in patients with chronic hyperandrogenic anovulation may have important therapeutic consequences.

REFERENCES

1. Stein, I.F. and Leventhal, M.L. (1935). Amenorrhea associated with bilateral polycystic ovaries. *Am. J. Obstet. Gynecol.*, **29**, 181–6
2. Goldzieher, J.W. and Axelrod, L.R. (1967). Clinical and biochemical features of polycystic ovarian disease. *Fertil. Steril.*, **14**, 631–53
3. Franks, S., Adams, J., Mason, H. and Polson, D. (1985). Ovulatory disorders in women with polycystic ovary syndrome. *Clin. Obstet. Gynecol.*, **12**, 605–32
4. Yen, S.S.C., Chaney, C. and Judd, H.L. (1976). Functional aberrations of the hypothalamic–pituitary system in polycystic ovary syndrome: a consideration of the pathogenesis. In James, V.H.T., Serio, M. and Giusti, G. (eds.) *The Endocrine Function of the Human Ovary*, pp. 373–85. (New York: Academic Press)
5. Givens, J.R. (1988). Familial polycystic ovarian disease. *Endocrinol. Metab. Clin. N. Am.*, **17**, 771–83
6. Jackson, A.S. and Pollock, M.L. (1985). Practical assessment of body composition. *Phys. Sportmed.*, **5**, 76–90
7. Ferriman, D. and Gallway, J.D. (1961). Clinical assessment of body hair growth in women. *J. Clin. Endocrinol. Metab.*, **21**, 1440–7
8. Eden, J.A., Place, J., Carter, G.D., Alaghband-Zadeh, J. and Pawson, M. (1989). Is the polycystic ovary a cause of infertility in the ovulatory woman? *Clin. Endocrinol.*, **30**, 77–82
9. Yen, S.S.C. (1980). The polycystic ovary syndrome. *Clin. Endocrinol.*, **12**, 177–208
10. Erickson, G.F., Hsueh, A.J.W., Quigley, M.E., Rebar, R.W. and Yen, S.S.C. (1979). Functional studies of aromatase activity in human granulosa cells from normal and polycystic ovaries. *J. Clin. Endocrinol. Metab.*, **49**, 514–19
11. Swanson, M., Sauerbrei, E.E. and Cooperberg, P.L. (1981). Medical implications of ultrasonically detected polycystic ovaries. *J. Clin. Ultrasound*, **9**, 219–22
12. Hann, L.E., Hall, D.A., McArdle, C.R. and Seibel, M. (1984). Polycystic ovary disease: sonographic spectrum. *Radiology.*, **150**, 531–4
13. Parisi, L., Tramonti, M., Derchi, L.E., Casciano, S., Zurli, A. and Rocchi, P. (1984). Polycystic ovarian disease: ultrasonic evaluation and correlations with clinical and hormonal data. *J. Clin. Ultrasound*, **12**, 21–6
14. Orsini, L.F., Venturoli, S., Lorusso, R., Pluchinotta, V., Paradisi, R. and Bovicelli, L. (1985). Ultrasonic findings in polycystic ovarian disease. *Fertil. Steril.*, **43**, 709–14
15. Adams, J., Polson, D.W. and Franks, S. (1986). Prevalence of polycystic ovaries in women with anovulation and idiopathic hirsutism. *Br. Med. J.*, **293**, 470–3
16. Tabbakh, G.H., Lofty, I., Azab, I., Rahman, H.A., Southren, A.L. and Aleem, F.A. (1986). Correlation of the ultrasonic appearance of the ovaries in polycystic ovarian disease and the clinical, hormonal, and laparoscopic findings. *Am. J. Obstet. Gynecol.*, **154**, 892–5
17. Yeh, H.-S., Futterweit, W. and Thornton, J.C. (1987). Polycystic ovarian disease: US features in 104 patients. *Radiology*, **163**, 111–16
18. Conway, G.S., Honour, J.W. and Jacobs, H.S. (1989). Heterogeneity of the polycystic ovary syndrome: clinical, endocrine and ultrasound features in 556 patients. *Clin. Endocrinol.*, **30**, 459–70

2

Structure of the polycystic ovary

S. Franks

INTRODUCTION

The ability to perform non-invasive imaging of the ovaries by pelvic ultrasonography has led to a reappraisal of the definition, diagnosis and prevalence of polycystic ovaries in women with hyperandrogenemia and anovulation. The following pages include a review of the histological features of the polycystic ovary, as judged by classic morphological examination, and a discussion of the role of ultrasound imaging of the ovaries in the investigation and management of women with polycystic ovary syndrome.

MORPHOLOGY: HISTOLOGICAL FEATURES

There have been numerous studies documenting the morphology of the polycystic ovary[1-8], but few have made a concerted attempt to quantitate the histological features which distinguish the polycystic from the normal ovary. Hughesdon[9], however, used both a descriptive and a quantitative approach to the analysis of ovarian tissue obtained after a full thickness transverse wedge resection. A summary of his findings in 34 polycystic compared with 30 normal ovaries is given in Table 1 and depicted in Figure 1. The polycystic ovaries were typically increased in size, although normal-sized ovaries with all the other characteristic histological features of polycystic ovaries were observed in his series. An important feature of the polycystic ovary was that, although the average number of primordial follicles was the

Table 1 Histological features of the polycystic compared with the normal ovary. Adapted from Hughesdon[9]

1   Increased volume (2 × cross-sectional area)
2   Same number of primordial follicles
3   Double the number of ripening and atretic follicles
4   Increased and more collagenized tunica
5   Slight increase in cortical stromal thickness
6   Greatly increased (5 ×) subcortical stroma with
      increased vascularity and innervation
7   Frequent occurrence of hilar cell nests

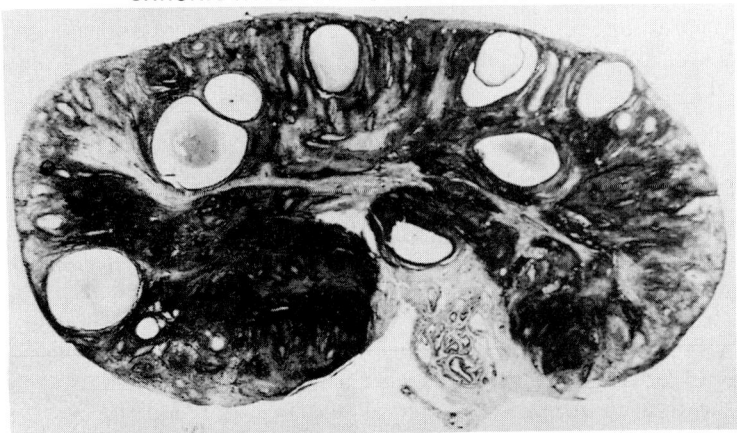

Figure 1 Section of a polycystic ovary showing many cystic follicles, thickened tunica with centripetal extensions and increased subcortical stroma. From Hughesdon[9] (with permission)

same as in a normal ovary, the number of ripening and atretic follicles was doubled. Thus all stages of folliculogenesis are increased in the polycystic ovary (Table 2) but the proportions of immature, mature and atretic follicles are similar to those observed in the normal ovary. There is a tendency for the tunica to be increased and to contain many collagen fibers. There is a slight increase in the cortical stroma but the subcortical stroma is greatly increased with the appearance of many small blood vessels and nerves, particularly in the hilar region. Small nests of hilar cells (which on electron microscopy show features of steroid-secreting cells) are also commonly found in the polycystic ovary[10].

The increased stroma which is so characteristic of the polycystic ovary appears to be derived primarily from atretic follicles. During atresia there is a striking hypertrophy of the theca cells[10] which then disperse into the interstitial tissue, often accumulating around small blood vessels[9]. It is the increased population of atretic follicles which accounts for the previously described 'theca cell hyperplasia', but it is important to realize that this is probably a normal function of atresia itself rather than an abnormality which affects developing follicles in the polycystic ovary. Primary mesenchymal hyperplasia may also contribute to the increase in stroma[9] but appears to play a lesser part in the genesis of the polycystic ovary than the theca-derived cells.

It remains unclear whether the increased androgen production from the polycystic ovary is simply a feature of the increased number of (luteinizing

Table 2 Ovarian cross-sectional area and follicle count in polycystic and control ovaries

	Size (cm^2)	*Primordial follicles*	*Follicle count**		
			Immature	*Mature*	*Atretic*
Polycystic ovaries	9.7	81	3.7	1.4	12.4
Normal	5.0	80	1.8	0.7	5.2

*Follicle count refers to the average number per section, adapted from Hughesdon[9]

hormone-responsive) theca-interstitial cells or whether the cells themselves are qualitatively different, in their steroidogenic capacity, from those in the normal ovary.

ULTRASOUND DIAGNOSIS OF POLYCYSTIC OVARIES

The increased number of follicles, and in particular the medium-sized to large antral follicles (2–10 mm in diameter) can be readily visualized using high resolution ultrasound scanning. Ultrasound will also demonstrate the increased stroma which typifies the polycystic ovary (Figure 2)[11–14]. The basis of the diagnosis (using the transabdominal route of scanning) is the finding of ten or more follicles, in one plane, together with increased stroma. Identification of increased stroma is relatively straightforward when the overall ovarian volume is increased (i.e. greater than 9 ml) but is more difficult to assess if the ovary is of normal volume. The appearance then has to be differentiated from that of the so-called multifollicular ovary[11]. The multifollicular ovary is observed during normal puberty and in women with mild or partially-recovered weight loss-related hypothalamic amenorrhea and is associated with a slowing of luteinizing hormone (LH) pulses[15]. In such cases the ovary is normal in size or slightly increased in volume and there is an increased number of follicles. However, the stroma is not increased and can be distinguished quite clearly from the normal-sized polycystic ovary (Figures 3 and 4). It is clear that transvaginal ultrasonography allows the definition of a larger number of small follicles than does transabdominal scanning even in the normal ovary. The criteria for the diagnosis of polycystic ovaries described above may need to be revised for the assessment of polycystic ovaries by vaginal ultrasonography.

CORRELATION OF ULTRASOUND WITH HISTOLOGY

It is important, when possible, to corroborate the findings on ultrasound by those on histology. In a recent study Saxton et al.[16] showed an excellent correlation between the morphological appearance as observed on ultrasound and that seen on histology. These observations lend confidence to the assertion that ultrasound can be reliably used for the diagnosis of polycystic ovaries.

PREVALENCE OF POLYCYSTIC OVARIES IN ANOVULATORY, HIRSUTE AND NORMAL SUBJECTS

We assessed the prevalence of polycystic ovaries in a population of patients attending a gynecological endocrine clinic with menstrual disturbances, hirsutism or both[14,17]. The prevalence of polycystic ovaries in these groups of women is summarized in Table 3. The vast majority of women with oligomenorrhea were found to have polycystic ovaries on ultrasound but,

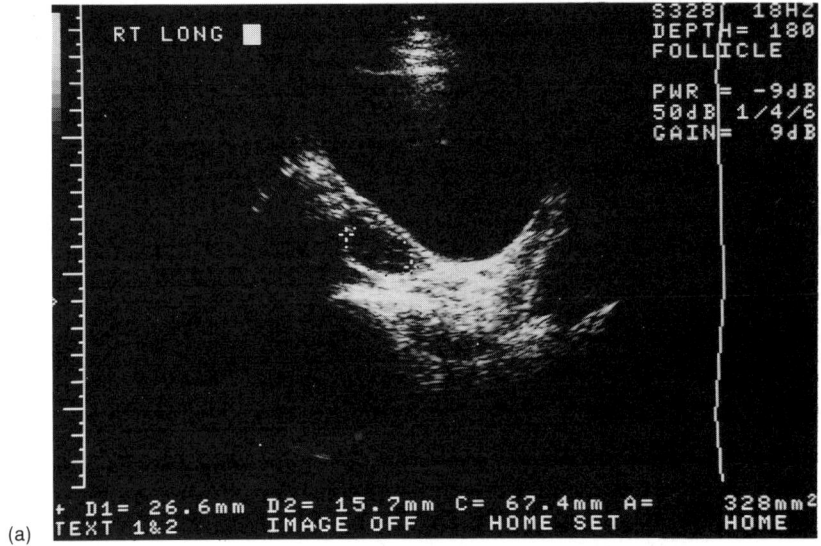

(a)

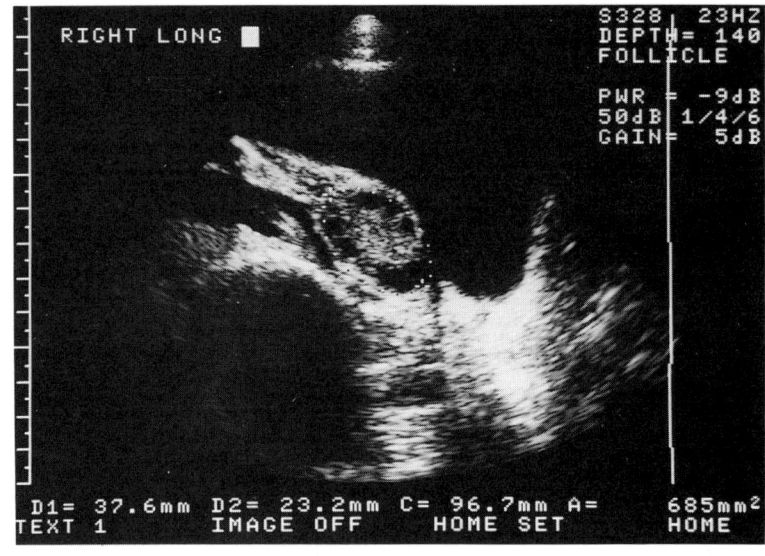

(b)

Figure 2 Transabdominal ultrasound scans showing longitudinal views of (a) normal and (b) polycystic ovary. Note increased size due to increased number of follicles and greater amount of stroma (pictures by courtesy of Miss D. Kiddy)

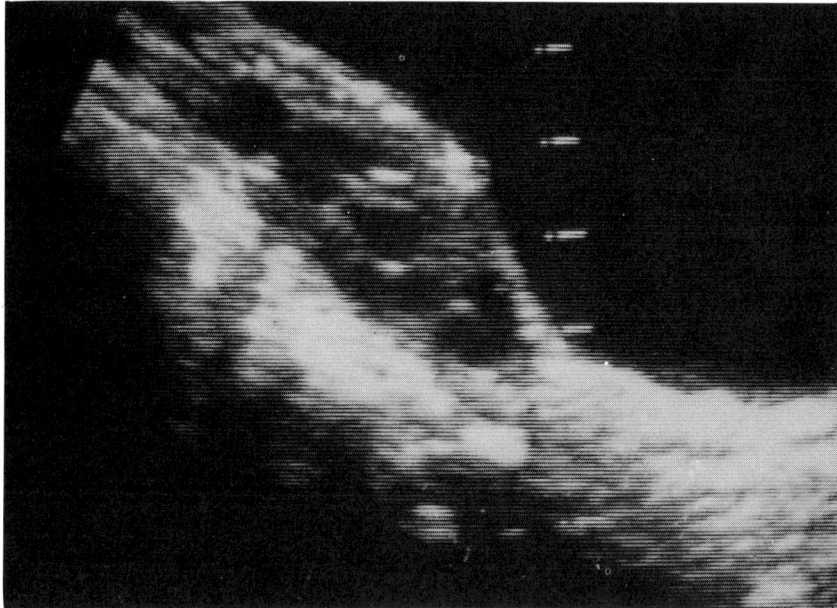

Figure 3 A multifollicular ovary in a normal girl in mid-puberty. This appearance is similar to that in women with weight loss-related hypothalamic amenorrhea. Note that the ovary is of normal size and is filled with follicles but that there is no increase in stroma (picture by courtesy of Miss J. Adams[23])

more surprisingly, those with regular ovulatory cycles who presented with hirsutism also had a high prevalence of polycystic ovaries. The appearance of polycystic ovaries in women with regular ovulatory cycles was an important finding since it suggests that the polycystic ovary represents a primary ovarian abnormality rather than the response of the ovary to chronic anovulation[17].

The endocrine evaluation of these three groups of women revealed that serum LH concentrations were significantly elevated compared with normal in all three groups, but that the levels in women with regular cycles and hirsutism were intermediate between normal subjects and those with anovulatory cycles (Table 3). A similar pattern was seen in serum testosterone. These endocrine features support the ultrasound diagnosis of polycystic ovaries. Subsequent results from a much larger series of subjects, in whom the primary diagnosis of polycystic ovary syndrome was made on ultrasound, have confirmed these initial endocrine findings[17].

Because of the high prevalence of polycystic ovaries in our population of patients we decided to examine a large group of volunteers from the normal population. All these women considered themselves to be normal and had not presented to a physician for treatment of menstrual disturbance or symptoms of hyperandrogenemia. We found that 22% of 257 women who presented for ultrasound scans had polycystic ovaries[18]. There was a strong correlation between the cycle history and the ovarian appearance (Table 4),

Normal **MFO** **PCO**

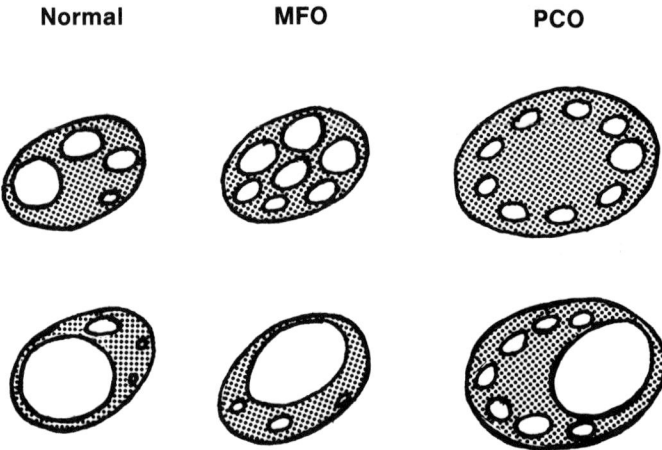

Figure 4 Diagnostic representation of a normal, multifollicular (MFO) and polycystic ovary (PCO) showing the change in appearance with the development of a dominant follicle. The presence of a dominant follicle in the multifollicular ovary is associated with normalization of the ovarian appearance, whereas in the polycystic ovary the multiple peripheral follicles remain, despite the presence of a preovulatory follicle

Table 3 Prevalence of polycystic ovaries (PCO) on ultrasound in women with anovulation and/or hirsutism. Hormone concentrations in women with PCO are compared with those in early–mid-follicular phase of subjects with normal ovaries and ovulatory cycles. LH results were compared by the Mann–Whitney U test and testosterone by Student's t test. Values of both LH and testosterone in each group of women with PCO were significantly greater ($p < 0.01$) than in normal controls

Presenting symptom	Prevalence of PCO (%)	LH (U/l)		Testosterone (nmol/l)	
		Median	Range	Mean	SD
Secondary amenorrhea	32	16.0	4.8–29	3.1	1.1
Oligomenorrhea	87	13.9	4.0–42	3.3	1.2
Hirsutism (regular cycle)	92	9.9	5.0–15	2.6	0.9
Normal controls	—	5.3	2.0–14	1.7	0.4

so that the majority of women in the normal population who had polycystic ovaries had slightly irregular cycles. Furthermore, although the mean and median serum LH concentrations in women with polycystic ovaries were no different from those in women with normal ovaries, there was a difference in the distribution of LH concentrations such that there was a preponderance of higher levels in those with polycystic ovaries[18].

These data suggest that the ovarian phenotype of the polycystic ovary is extremely common and other studies have suggested that it is genetic in origin[19,20]. Development of polycystic ovary syndrome probably depends

Table 4 Correlation of ovarian appearance on ultrasound with menstrual history in the normal population

Ultrasound appearance	Regular menses	Irregular menses
Normal ovaries	115	1
Polycystic ovaries	8*	24

*Six of eight women with PCO and regular cycles were hirsute

on the interaction of other genetic and environmental factors (e.g. obesity) which affect the clinical and biochemical expression of the disorder[17,18,21].

FUNCTIONAL MORPHOLOGY OF THE POLYCYSTIC OVARY

The endocrine abnormalities described above give some indication of the abnormal function of the polycystic ovary and this subject will be dealt with in detail in the following chapter. So far, little is known about the cellular function of the theca interstitial cells which give rise to the characteristically elevated serum androgen concentrations[22]. There may, however, be important differences in the functional capacity of the ovarian stromal cells in polycystic compared with normal ovaries but, as mentioned above, it remains to be determined whether the interstitial cell is the site of the primary disorder in the polycystic ovary or whether it is secondary to a factor or factors which stimulate the increase in folliculogenesis[9,10].

REFERENCES

1. Allen, W.M. and Woolf, R.B. (1959). Medullary resection of the ovaries in the Stein–Leventhal syndrome. *Am. J. Obstet. Gynecol.*, **77**, 826–34
2. Goldzieher, J.W. and Green, J.A. (1962). The polycystic ovary. I. Clinical and histologic features. *J. Clin. Endocrinol. Metab.*, **22**, 325–38
3. Green, J.A. and Goldzieher, J.W. (1965). The polycystic ovary. IV. Light and electron microscopic studies. *Am. J. Obstet. Gynecol.*, **91**, 173–81
4. Ingersoll, F.M. and McDermott, W.V. (1950). Bilateral polycystic ovaries, Stein–Leventhal syndrome. *Am. J. Obstet. Gynecol.*, **60**, 117–25
5. Leventhal, M.L. (1958). The Stein–Leventhal syndrome. *Am. J. Obstet. Gynecol.*, **76**, 825–38
6. Plate, W.P. (1958). The pathologic anatomy of the Stein–Leventhal syndrome. *Fertil. Steril.*, **9**, 545–54
7. Shippel, S. (1955). The ovarian theca cell. IV. The hyperthecosis syndrome. *J. Obstet. Gynaecol. Br. Emp.*, **62**, 321–53
8. Westman, A. (1955). The histology and structure of the ovary in cases of virilism. *Acta Obstet. Gynecol. Scand.*, **34**, 92–104
9. Hughesdon, P.E. (1982). Morphology and morphogenesis of the Stein–Leventhal ovary and of so-called 'hyperthecosis'. *Obstet. Gynecol. Surv.*, **37**, 59–77
10. Erickson, G.F., Magoffin, D.A., Dyer, C.A. and Hofeditz, C. (1985). The ovarian androgen producing cells: a review of structure/function relationships. *Endocrine Rev.*, **6**, 371–99
11. Swanson, M., Sauerbrei, E.E. and Cooperberg, P.L. (1981). Medical implications of ultrasonically detected polycystic ovaries. *J. Clin. Ultrasound*, **9**, 219–22

12. Parisi, L., Tramonti, M., Casciano, S., Zurli, A. and Gazzarrini, O. (1982). The role of ultrasound in the study of polycystic ovarian disease. *J. Clin. Ultrasound*, **10**, 167–72
13. Adams, J., Franks, S., Polson, D.W., Mason, H.D., Abdulwahid, N.A., Tucker, M., Morris, D.V., Price, J. and Jacobs, H.S. (1985). Multifollicular ovaries: clinical and endocrine features and response to pulsatile gonadotrophin releasing hormone. *Lancet*, **2**, 1375–8
14. Adams, J., Polson, D.W. and Franks, S. (1986). Prevalence of polycystic ovaries in women with anovulation and idiopathic hirsutism. *Br. Med. J.*, **293**, 355–9
15. Mason, H.D., Sagle, M., Polson, D.W., Kiddy, D., Dobriansky, D., Adams, J. and Franks, S. (1988). Reduced frequency of luteinizing hormone pulses in women with weight loss-related amenorrhoea and multifollicular ovaries. *Clin. Endocrinol.*, **28**, 611–18
16. Saxton, D.W., Farquhar, C.M., Rae, T., Beard, R.W., Anderson, M.C. and Wadsworth, J. (1990). Accuracy of ultrasound measurements of female pelvic organs. *Br. J. Obstet. Gynaecol.*, in press
17. Franks, S. (1989). Polycystic ovary syndrome: a changing perspective. *Clin. Endocrinol.*, **31**, 87–120
18. Polson, D.W., Adams, J., Wadsworth, J. and Franks, S. (1988). Polycystic ovaries – a common finding in normal women. *Lancet*, **1**, 870–2
19. Wilroy, R.S., Givens, J.R., Wiser, W.L., Coleman, S.A., Andersen, R.N. and Summitt, R.L. (1975). Hyperthecosis: an inheritable form of polycystic ovarian disease. *Birth Defects*, original article: Series XI, 81–5
20. Hague, W., Adams, J., Reeders, S., Peto, T.E.A. and Jacobs, H.S. (1988). Familial polycystic ovaries: a genetic disease. *Clin. Endocrinol.*, **29**, 593–606
21. Kiddy, D.S., Hamilton-Fairley, D., Seppala, M., Koistinen, R., James, V.H.T., Reed, M.J. and Franks, S. (1989). Diet-induced changes in sex hormone-binding globulin and free testosterone in women with normal or polycystic ovaries: correlation with serum insulin and insulin-like growth factor-I. *Clin. Endocrinol.*, **31**, 757–63
22. Barbieri, R.L., Makris, A., Randall, R.W., Daniels, G., Kistner, R.W. and Ryan, K.J. (1986). Insulin stimulates androgen accumulation in incubations of ovarian stroma obtained from women with hyperandrogenism. *J. Clin. Endocrinol. Metab.*, **62**, 904–9
23. Stanhope, R., Adams, J., Jacobs, H.S. and Brook, C.G.D. (1985). Ovarian ultrasound assessment in normal children, idiopathic precocious puberty and during low dose pulsatile GnRH therapy of hypogonadotrophic hypogonadism. *Arch. Dis. Child.*, **60**, 116–19

3

Follicular function in polycystic ovaries

S.G. Hillier

INTRODUCTION

Polycystic ovary syndrome (PCOS) and related forms of chronic hyper-androgenic anovulation are major causes of infertility in women. Endocrino-logically, they are characterized by circulating plasma gonadotropin levels which do not show normal cyclic patterns consistent with ovulation, and chronically elevated circulating androgen levels. Classically, the luteinizing hormone (LH) level is abnormally high in the face of a low to normal follicle stimulating hormone (FSH) level (see ref. 1 for review). This article analyzes the regulatory actions of FSH and LH on follicular development in ovulatory menstrual cycles, as a basis for understanding the impacts of understimulation by FSH and overstimulation by LH on the development of hyperandrogenic, anovulatory ovarian function in PCOS.

FSH FUNCTION AND PREOVULATORY FOLLICULAR DEVELOPMENT

Intercyclic increases in blood FSH provide the endocrine stimulus for preovulatory follicular development in spontaneous ovulatory cycles[2]. FSH acts directly to stimulate cell proliferation and cytodifferentiation in the granulosa layer of follicles of around 5 mm in diameter at the beginning of the follicular phase. Hallmarks of FSH action are increased follicular steroid (estradiol) and secretory protein (inhibin) synthesis, associated with increased responsiveness to FSH and LH (see refs. 3–5 for reviews).

Mechanism of FSH action

Granulosa cells are the only ovarian cells which possess FSH receptors. FSH binding to its receptor on the cell surface activates intracellular adenylyl cyclase and cyclic AMP-dependent protein kinase(s), leading to expression of genes encoding the proteins which coordinate granulosa cell growth and differentiation[6].

Granulosa cell aromatase activity

Expression of aromatase activity is the primary steroidogenic marker of granulosa cell differentiation. This FSH-induced cytochrome P450 steroidogenic enzyme catalyzes the final rate-limiting step in estrogen biosynthesis, using androgenic precursors produced by the LH-stimulated theca interna (see below). During the mid–late follicular phase of the cycle, the estrogen-secretory follicle which is destined to ovulate is recognizable by its highly active granulosa cell aromatase system and proportionately elevated follicular fluid estrogen level[7]. Besides its classic endocrine function, follicular estrogen serves local regulatory functions. Experiments in rats have shown that estrogen stimulates granulosa cell proliferation and augments granulosa cell responsiveness to FSH and LH[3–6]. The mechanism and functional significance of regulatory estrogen action in human granulosa cells are uncertain. However, using the common marmoset as a non-human primate model, it has been shown that estradiol augments FSH-induced granulosa cell inhibin production *in vitro*[8]. This is potentially important since inhibins and related proteins may also serve functions in the ovarian paracrine system[9,10].

Granulosa cell responsiveness to FSH

The preovulatory follicle has a diminished requirement for stimulation by FSH during the late follicular phase of the ovarian cycle[11]. Thus the aromatase activity of granulosa cells isolated from the preovulatory follicle is many times higher and more sensitive to FSH than that of granulosa cells from immature follicles[12].

Granulosa cell responsiveness to LH

Granulosa cells also acquire increased responsiveness to LH during advanced preovulatory follicular development[3–6]. Experiments with human and non-human primate ovarian tissues have shown that granulosa cells from preovulatory follicles express an LH-responsive aromatase system, which is absent in the granulosa cells from immature follicles[13]. The key to this change is the induction by FSH of granulosa cell LH receptors[3–5].

Granulosa cell responsiveness to gonadotropins and selection of the dominant follicle

The induction by FSH of FSH- and LH-responsive granulosa cell aromatase activity is central to the mechanism whereby a single estrogen-secretory follicle develops and ovulates in the human menstrual cycle. When the plasma FSH level rises at the beginning of each cycle, the ovaries contain multiple follicles around 5 mm in diameter with varying potentials for FSH-dependent development. Each follicle present requires a different degree of stimulation by FSH for it to undergo preovulatory development. The follicle which eventually grows to a diameter of over 20 mm or so and ovulates is thought to be the one whose granulosa cells most rapidly acquire high levels of aromatase and LH receptor in response to the intercycle FSH rise, i.e. the one with the lowest FSH 'threshold'[14,15]. During the midfollicular phase, estradiol secretion by this follicle begins to increase and the steroid feeds back to negatively regulate pituitary FSH secretion. This causes a progressive reduction in the circulating FSH level and thereby limits FSH-dependent development of other follicles with relatively high 'threshold' FSH requirements. Thus only one follicle becomes fully mature, protected against the fall in circulating FSH by its high responsiveness to both FSH and LH[12]. Local actions of estrogen within the dominant follicle may further enhance its gonadotropin-responsiveness, as discussed above.

CONSEQUENCES OF INADEQUATE OVARIAN STIMULATION BY FSH IN PCOS

Measurements of immuno-[1] and bioactive[16] FSH levels in serial daily blood samples have shown that the early follicular phase and mid-cycle FSH peaks, which characterize ovulatory menstrual cycles, are absent in PCOS. This appears to be the major reason why the follicles present in polycystic ovaries do not undergo advanced stages of preovulatory development[17].

FSH-dependent granulosa cell function in PCOS

Studies of FSH-dependent granulosa cell function have been undertaken using cells recovered from the follicles in wedge biopsies from polycystic ovaries[17]. Results show that granulosa cells from PCOS follicles evince 'normal' FSH-responsiveness, based on measurements of aromatase activity *in vitro*. PCOS follicles seem to fall into two categories: relatively small follicles ≤ 5 mm in diameter, which are morphologically healthy and yield FSH-responsive granulosa cells; and larger follicles which are more likely to be undergoing atresia. Granulosa cells from < 5 mm diameter PCOS follicles have higher levels of basal and FSH-responsive aromatase activity compared with those from larger follicles in the same wedge (Hillier, S.G., unpublished observation).

Follicular fluid estrogen levels in PCOS

Estrogen levels in PCOS follicular fluid are low, similar to those in fluid from follicles of a similar size in normal ovaries[18]. This is consistent with the lack of estrogen-secretory preovulatory follicle development in polycystic ovaries.

Functional FSH inadequacy as the basis of anovulation in PCOS

An ovulatory menstrual cycle can often be induced in a PCOS patient by treatment with exogenous FSH[19]. This, combined with evidence that granulosa cells from many of the follicles in polycystic ovaries can respond normally to treatment with FSH *in vitro*, suggests that inappropriate ovarian stimulation by FSH is the major cause of chronic anovulation in PCOS. The cortical region of polycystic ovaries is typically packed with follicles similar in size and morphology to the largest healthy follicles which are present in 'normal' ovaries at the beginning of an ovulatory menstrual cycle (i.e. around 5 mm in diameter)[16,18,20,21]. However, in PCOS, the ovaries do not receive the intercyclic FSH signal required to initiate preovulatory follicular development. In the absence of this signal, FSH-dependent follicular development ceases. Thus granulosa cells do not acquire a fully activated aromatase system and remain unresponsive to LH. Estrogen biosynthesis is suppressed and atresia sets in. This explains why most of the relatively large follicles in polycystic ovaries are degenerate.

LH FUNCTION AND PREOVULATORY FOLLICULAR DEVELOPMENT

Ovarian stimulation by LH is required to maintain the development of the theca interna in follicles at all stages of antral development. The theca interna regulated by LH is the major follicular site of androgen synthesis. Secondary interstitial cells derived from the thecae of degenerated follicles are also sites of LH-regulated androgen synthesis in the stroma (see ref. 22 for review).

LH mechanism of action

LH receptors are located on thecal/interstitial cells and androgen synthesis at these sites is under direct LH control throughout the menstrual cycle. LH acts via its receptor on thecal cells to activate adenylyl cyclase signalling, which increases precursor-cholesterol uptake and sustains the C17-hydroxylase/C-17,20 lyase functions of cytochrome $P450_{17}$, the rate-limiting enzyme in androgen synthesis[22].

Thecal control of granulosa cell function

During normal preovulatory follicular development, androgens (androstenedione and testosterone) synthesized in the LH-stimulated theca are used by granulosa cells as precursors for estrogen synthesis[23]. The granulosa cell aromatase system induced by FSH during the first half of the follicular phase becomes directly responsive to LH during the second half of the follicular phase (see above).

The 'two-cell, two gonadotropin' mechanism explains how theca and granulosa cells interact to synthesize estrogen[23] and highlights the manner whereby the theca imposes local regulatory control over granulosa cell function via paracrine signalling[5]. During earlier stages of preovulatory follicular development, before granulosa cells acquire LH receptors, androgens and possibly non-steroidal factors produced by LH-stimulated thecal cells appear to modulate granulosa cell responsiveness to FSH. There is increasing evidence that androgens[5] and transforming growth factor β (TGF-β)[24,25] may function as positive paracrine factors which promote the expression of FSH-inducible function (steroidogenesis and protein secretion) during early antral stages of follicular development. Other thecal non-steroidal factors, including TGF-α, are implicated in the regulation of granulosa cell replication and may inhibit the expression of differentiated granulosa cell function[26,27]. Although LH is a major factor in the control of thecal androgen synthesis, its role in regulating non-steroidal paracrine signalling by the theca interna remains to be established.

Thecal androgens augment FSH-inducible granulosa cell function via amplification of cyclic AMP-mediated intracellular signalling. Many FSH-dependent granulosa cell functions, including steroidogenesis, inhibin production and expression of LH receptors, are susceptible to augmentation by androgens in this way[5].

The stimulatory effects of androgen on FSH-dependent granulosa cell function diminish as the cells differentiate and acquire direct responsiveness to LH. During advanced preovulatory development androgen becomes ineffective or inhibitory. Thus, whereas induction by FSH of aromatase activity in granulosa cells from immature follicles is markedly augmented by testosterone and 5α-dihydrotestosterone *in vitro*, these androgens suppress the stimulatory effect of FSH on aromatase activity in more mature granulosa cells[13].

Naturally occurring 5α-reduced androgen metabolites such as 5α-dihydrotestosterone and androsterone are competitive inhibitors of the granulosa cell aromatase reaction *in vitro*[28]. Small quantities of these 5α-reduced androgens are present in human ovarian follicular fluid[29] and 5α-reductase activity is present in both theca and granulosa cells[30]. However, nothing is known about the regulation of this enzymic activity or its functional significance in human ovaries. Whether 5α-reduced androgens play significant roles as competitive inhibitors of aromatization or as paracrine regulators of granulosa cell function *in vivo* is also uncertain.

IMPLICATIONS OF EXCESSIVE OVARIAN STIMULATION BY LH IN PCOS

The hyperandrogenic state in PCOS is due to increased androgen secretion by the ovaries and adrenal glands[31,32]. The ovarian contribution is secondary to increased pulsatile release of LH by the pituitary gland and excessive stimulation of the ovaries by LH[1]. Polycystic ovaries contain relatively abundant amounts of hypertrophied stromal interstitial tissue (hyperthecosis) as compared with 'normal' ovaries, and the thecae of the multiple follicles which are present may display variable degrees of hypertrophy[20]. The hyperthecosis is caused by an increased accumulation of secondary interstitial tissue due to the relatively high rate of follicular atresia which occurs in polycystic ovaries. It is doubtful if the thecae of individual PCOS follicles undertake excessive rates of androgen synthesis as compared with the thecae of 'normal' follicles at equivalent stages of development[33,34]. However, stromal androgen production is increased in PCOS ovaries[34]. Thus, chronic stimulation by LH combined with the overall increased amount of androgen-secretory stromal and thecal tissue present are major reasons for the excessive rate of ovarian androgen secretion in PCOS.

Insulin may also augment androgen production by polycystic ovaries. This is suggested by the strong relationship between hyperandrogenism and hyperinsulinism[35], the presence of insulin receptors in stromal and thecal tissue[36], and the demonstration that insulin can stimulate stromal androgen production *in vitro*[37]. Insulin-like growth factor-1 (IGF-1) also stimulates stromal androgen production *in vitro*[37]. However, IGF-1 levels in follicular fluid from PCOS do not appear to differ significantly from those in 'normal' follicular fluids[38].

Follicular fluid androgen levels in PCOS

Androgen levels in PCOS follicular fluids are either slightly elevated[18] or within the ranges observed for normal and atretic follicles of equivalent sizes in 'normal' ovaries[30]. 5α-reduced androgens (potential aromatase inhibitors: see above) are present in follicular fluid from polycystic ovaries but they do not appear to exceed the levels present in 'normal' follicular fluids[32,34]. However, it is difficult to know what constitutes an appropriate control against which to assess the steroid content of PCOS follicular fluid, since marked interfollicular differences in androgen levels exist among follicles of a similar size in 'normal' ovaries[21].

Negative regulation of granulosa cell development by thecal androgens

The granulosa cell layer is literally drenched in androgen throughout most of the preovulatory follicle's antral stages of follicular development in 'normal' ovaries[5]; therefore it is difficult to invoke a negative regulatory action of androgen which is peculiar to PCOS. However, from basic experimental work with hypophysectomized immature female rats (reviewed in ref. 5), it is known that treatment with androgen or LH (without FSH) interferes with the limited development of the preantral follicles which persist after hypophysectomy. Moreover, estrogen given alone increases preantral follicular development and this effect is inhibited by co-treatment with androgen or LH. Thus, in the absence of FSH, androgen promotes follicular atresia in rat ovaries. Given the functionally inadequate FSH status of PCOS patients, excessive intraovarian androgen levels would also seem likely to exacerbate follicular atresia in polycystic ovaries.

CONCLUDING REMARKS

Anovulation in most forms of polycystic ovary syndrome appears to be due to a quantitative deficiency in the circulating FSH level needed to promote degrees of granulosa cell proliferation and differentiation consistent with normal preovulatory follicular development. Healthy follicles in polycystic ovaries rarely develop beyond a diameter of about 5 mm because their granulosa cell aromatase systems do not become fully activated and LH receptors are not expressed. These follicles cease to develop normally and eventually become atretic because their granulosa cells are unable to synthesize adequate amounts of estrogen or respond directly to LH.

Chronic ovarian hyperstimulation by LH, compounded by hyperinsulinemia in many cases is a primary cause of hyperandrogenism in polycystic ovary syndrome. Ovarian rates of aromatizable and non-aromatizable androgen secretion are enhanced in polycystic ovary syndrome but it is not clear if they are due to LH-stimulated increases in androgen synthesis within the thecae of individual follicles or to a net increase in the overall number of androgen secretory atretic follicles which accumulates. However, the increased rate of follicular atresia results in the build up of secondary interstitial tissue in the ovarian stroma (hyperthecosis) which is a major site of excessive androgen synthesis in polycystic ovaries.

In the absence of appropriate stimulation by FSH, follicular androgens produced by LH-stimulated thecal cells inhibit granulosa cell function, further increasing the incidence of follicular atresia. Thecal non-steroidal factors may also suppress granulosa cell responsiveness to FSH. It seems unlikely that the paracrine factors which affect granulosa cell function in polycystic ovaries are quantitatively or qualitatively different from those which regulate granulosa cell function in 'normal' ovaries.

REFERENCES

1. Yen, S.S.C. (1986). Chronic anovulation caused by peripheral endocrine disorders. In Yen, S.S.C. and Jaffe, R.B. (eds.) *Reproductive Endocrinology*, 2nd edn. pp. 441–99. (Philadelphia and London: W.B. Saunders)
2. Ross, G.T., Cargille, C.M., Lipsett, M.B. *et al.* (1970). Pituitary and gonadal hormones in women with spontaneous and induced ovulatory cycles. *Rec. Prog. Horm. Res.*, **26**, 1–62
3. Richards, J.S. (1980). Maturation of ovarian follicles: action and interaction of pituitary and ovarian hormones on follicular differentiation. *Physiol. Rev.*, **60**, 51–89
4. Hsueh, A.J.W., Adashi, E.Y., Jones, P.B.C. and Welsh, T.J. Jr. (1984). Hormonal regulation of the differentiation of cultured granulosa cells. *Endocr. Rev.*, **5**, 76–127
5. Hillier, S.G. (1985). Sex steroid metabolism and follicular development in the ovaries. In Clarke, J.R. (ed.) *Oxford Reviews of Reproductive Biology*, Vol. 7, pp. 168–222. (Oxford: Clarendon Press)
6. Richards, J.S., Jahnsen, T., Hedin, L., Lifka, J., Ratoosh, S.L., Durica, J.M. and Goldring, N.B. (1987). Ovarian follicular development: from physiology to molecular biology. *Rec.*

Prog. Horm. Res., **43**, 231–70

7. Hillier, S.G., Reichert, L.E.R. Jr. and van Hall, E.V. (1981). Control of preovulatory follicular estrogen biosynthesis in the human ovary. *J. Clin. Endocrinol. Metab.*, **52**, 847–56

8. Hillier, S.G., Wickings, E.J., Saunders, P.T.K.S., Dixson, A.F., Shimasaki, S., Swanston, I.A., Reichert, L.E. Jr. and McNeilly, A.S. (1989). Control of inhibin production by primate granulosa cells. *J. Endocrinol.*, **123**, 65–73

9. Bicsak, T.A. and Hsueh, A.J.W. (1987). Recent advances in inhibin research. In Stouffer, R.L. (ed.) *The Primate Ovary*, pp. 35–47. (New York and London: Plenum Press)

10. Turner, I.M., Sanders, P.T.K.S., Shimasaki, S. and Hillier, S.G. (1989). Regulation of inhibin subunit gene expression of FSH and estradiol in cultured rat granulosa cells. *Endocrinology*, **125**, in press

11. Zeleznik, A.J. and Kubik, C.J. (1986). Ovarian responses in macaques to pulsatile infusion of follicle-stimulating hormone (FSH) and luteinizing hormone: increased sensitivity of the maturing follicle. *Endocrinology*, **119**, 2025–32

12. Harlow, C.R., Shaw, H.J., Hillier, S.G. and Hodges, J.K. (1988). Factors influencing follicle-stimulating hormone-responsive steroidogenesis in marmoset granulosa cells. Effects of androgens and the stage of follicular maturity. *Endocrinology*, **122**, 2780–7

13. Shaw, H.J., Hillier, S.G. and Hodges, J.K. (1989). Developmental changes in luteinizing hormone/human chorionic gonadotropin steroidogenic responsiveness in marmoset granulosa cells: effects of follicle-stimulating hormone and androgens. *Endocrinology*, **124**, 1669–77

14. Brown, J.B. (1978). Pituitary control of ovarian function – concepts derived from gonadotrophin therapy. *Aust. N.Z.J. Obstet. Gynaecol.*, **18**, 47–54

15. Hillier, S.G. (1981). Regulation of follicular oestrogen biosynthesis: a survey of current concepts. *J. Endocrinol.*, **89**, 3P–18P

16. Reddi, K., Wickings, E.J. Hillier, S.G. and Baird, D.T. (1989). Bioactive FSH and inhibin concentrations during ovulation induction in patients with polycystic ovarian disease. *J. Endocrinol.*, **123**, (Suppl.), abstr.

17. Erickson, G.F., Hsueh, A.J., Quigley, M.E., Rebar, R.W. and Yen, S.S.C. (1979). Functional studies of aromatase activity in human granulosa cells from normal and polycystic ovaries. *J. Clin. Endocrinol. Metab.*, **49**, 514–19

18. Tanabe, K., Galiano, P., Channing, C.P., Nakamura, Y., Yoshimura, Y., Iizuka, R., Fortuny, A., Sulewski, J. and Rezai, N. (1983). Levels of inhibin-F activity and steroids in human follicular fluid from normal women and women with polycystic ovarian disease. *J. Clin. Endocrinol. Metab.*, **57**, 24–31

19. Coney, P. (1984). Polycystic ovarian disease: current concepts of pathophysiology and therapy. *Fertil. Steril.*, **42**, 667–82

20. Hughesdon, P.E. (1982). Morphology and morphogenesis of the Stein–Leventhal ovary and of so-called 'hyperthecosis'. *Obstet. Gynecol. Surv.*, **37**, 59–77

21. McNatty, K.P., Hillier, S.G., van den Boogaard, A.M.J., Trimbos-Kemper, T.C.M., Reichert, L.E. Jr. and van Hall, E.V. (1983). Follicular development during the luteal phase of the human menstrual cycle. *J. Clin. Endocrinol. Metab.*, **56**, 1022–31

22. Erickson, G.F. (1985). The ovarian androgen producing cells: a review of structure/function relationships. *Endocr. Rev.*, **6**, 371–99

23. Armstrong, D.T. and Dorrington, J.H. (1979). Estrogen biosynthesis in the ovaries and testes. In Thomas, J.A. and Singhal, R.L. (eds.) *Regulatory Mechanisms Affecting Gonadal Hormone Action*, Vol. 2, pp. 217–58. (Baltimore: University Park Press)

24. Skinner, M.K., Keski-Oja, J., Osteen, K.G. and Moses, H.L. (1987). Ovarian theca cells produce transforming growth factor-b which can regulate granulosa cell growth. *Endocrinology*, **121**, 786–92

25. Schomberg, D.W. (1987). Regulation of follicle development by gonadotropins and growth factors. In Stouffer, R.L. (ed.) *The Primate Ovary*, pp. 25–33. (New York and London: Plenum Press)

26. May, J.V., Frost, J.P. and Schomberg, D.W. (1988). Differential effects of epidermal growth factor, somatomedin-C/insulin-like growth factor I, and transforming growth factor-β on porcine granulosa cell deoxyribonucleic acid synthesis and cell proliferation. *Endocrinology*, **123**, 168–79

27. Kudlow, J.E., Korbrin, M.S., Purchio, A.F., Twardzik, D.R., Hernandez, E.R., Asa, S.L. and

Adashi, E.Y. (1987). Ovarian transforming growth factor-α gene expression: immunohisto-chemical localization to the theca-intersitial cells. *Endocrinology*, **121**, 1577–9

28. Hillier, S.G., van den Boogaard, A.J.M., Reichert, L.E. Jr. and van Hall, E.V. (1980). Intraovarian sex steroid hormone interactions and the control of follicular maturation: aromatization of androgens by human granulosa cells *in vitro*. *J. Clin. Endocrinol. Metab.*, **50**, 640–7

29. Dehennin, L., Jondet, L. and Scholler, R. (1987). Androgen and 19-norsteroid profiles in human preovulatory follicles from stimulated cycles: an isotope dilution–mass spectrometric study. *J. Steroid Biochem.*, **26**, 399–405

30. McNatty, K.P., Reinhold, V.N., DeGrazia, C., Osathanondh, R. and Ryan, K. (1979). Metabolism of androstenedione by human ovarian tissue *in vitro* with particular reference to reductase and aromatase activity. *Steroids*, **34**, 429–43

31. Kirschner, M.A. and Jacobs, J.B. (1971). Combined adrenal and ovarian vein catheterization to determine the site(s) of androgen overproduction in hirsute women. *J. Clin. Endocrinol. Metab.*, **33**, 199–209

32. Laatikainen, T.J., Apter, D.L., Paavonen, J.A. and Wahlstrom, T.R. (1980). Steroids in ovarian and peripheral venous blood in polycystic ovarian disease. *Clin. Endocrinol. (Oxf.)*, **13**, 125–34

33. Wilson, E.A., Erickson, G.F., Zarutski, P., Finn, A.E., Tulchinsky, D. and Ryan, K.J. (1979). Endocrine studies of normal and polycystic ovarian tissues *in vitro*. *Am. J. Obstet. Gynecol.*, **134**, 56–63

34. McNatty, K.P., Smith, D.W., Makris, A., DeGrazia, C., Tulchinsky, D., Osathanondh, R., Schiff, I. and Ryan, K.J. (1980). The intraovarian sites of androgen and estrogen formation in women with normal and hyperandrogenic ovaries as judged by *in vitro* experiments. *J. Clin. Endocrinol. Metab.*, **50**, 755–64

35. Chang, R.J., Nakamura, R.M., Judd, H.L. and Kaplan, S.A. (1983). Insulin resistance in nonobese patients with polycystic ovarian disease. *J. Clin. Endocrinol. Metab.*, **57**, 356–9

36. Poretsky, L., Grigorescu, F., Seibel, M., Moses, A.C. and Flier, J.S. (1985). Distribution and characterization of insulin and insulin-like growth factor receptors in normal human ovary. *J. Clin. Endocrinol. Metab.*, **61**, 728–34

37. Barbieri, R.L., Makris, A., Randall, R.W., Daniels, G., Kistner, R.W. and Ryan, K.J. (1986). Insulin stimulates androgen accumulation in incubations of ovarian stroma obtained from women with hyperandrogenism. *J. Clin. Endocrinol. Metab.*, **62**, 904–10

38. Eden, J.A., Jones, J., Carter, G.D. and Alaghband-Zadeh, J. (1988). A comparison of follicular fluid levels of insulin-like growth factor-I in normal dominant and cohort follicles, polycystic and multicystic ovaries. *Clin. Endocrinol. (Oxf.)*, **29**, 327–36

4

The hypothalamic–pituitary unit in chronic hyperandrogenism: potential for management by development of a GnRH antagonist (ORG 30850)

*K. Gordon, R.T. Scott, R.F. Williams, D.R. Danforth,
H.J.J. Loozen, H.J. Kloosterboer and G.D. Hodgen*

INTRODUCTION

This chapter is developed in two parts. The first part reviews some of the etiologic and pathophysiologic derangements of hypothalamic–pituitary function commonly associated with chronic hyperandrogenism (CHA). The second part is devoted to recent findings on the potential usefulness of a gonadotropin releasing hormone (GnRH) antagonist (ORG 30850) to suppress the secretion of gonadotropins, inhibit ovarian steroidogenesis, and serve adjunctively with either gonadotropin therapy or GnRH pulsatile administration to achieve ovulation induction (Scott, R.T. *et al.*, unpublished data).

ETIOLOGIC AND PATHOPHYSIOLOGIC DERANGEMENTS

The classical study by Goldzieher and Axelrod[1] set forth an estimate of the frequency of various hormonal, metabolic and phenotypic aberrations among women having CHA (also known as polycystic ovary syndrome) (Table 1). The CHA hormonal deviations occurring often include:

(1) Elevated androgens;

(2) Supranormal luteinizing hormone (LH), with follicle stimulating hormone (FSH) either normal or slightly below normal; and

(3) Excessive estrone (E_1), whereas estradiol (E_2) may be normal to low; however, typically, these patients are not hypoestrogenic[2,3].

Since CHA manifests as a spectrum of these hormonal aberrations in

Table 1 Symptomatology associated with surgically proven cases of polycystic ovary syndrome (from Goldzieher and Axelrod[1])

Symptom	Usable number of cases	Incidence Mean (%)	Range (%)
Obesity	600	41	16–49
Hirsutism	819	69	17–83
Virilization	431	21	0–28
Cyclic menses	395	12	7–28
Functional bleeding	547	29	6–25
Amenorrhea	640	51	15–77
Dysmenorrhea	75	23	—
Biphasic basal body temperature	238	15	12–40
Corpus luteum at operation	391	22	0–71
Infertility	596	74	35–94

various degrees, the etiology and pathophysiology do not fit into clear and obvious delineations. For example, whereas the excessive levels of androgens in circulation, in association with chronic oligo-ovulation, irregularities of the menstrual cycle and hirsutism, are the principal basis for calling the syndrome CHA, the overproduction of androgens may derive from ovarian or adrenal tissues or both, and proceed in parallel with obesity and abnormalities of carbohydrate and/or lipid metabolism.

The specific derangements of gonadotropin secretion may have subtle origins. Typically, the hypothalamus emits pulsatile GnRH and, in turn, the pituitary secretes a clearly pulsatile pattern of LH and FSH. However, increasing evidence points to an exaggeration of the amplitude of LH release per pulse, perhaps without irregularities of pulse frequency (Figure 1)[4]. It has been postulated that CHA begins with the onset of puberty itself, if not even earlier during adrenarche. Whatever the true etiologic mechanism(s), the emergence of what may be termed 'the vicious circle' ensues rapidly in the reproductive life of young women manifesting the clinical symptoms of CHA (Figure 2)[5]. Whether inhibin or other non-steroidal gonadal factors contribute to CHA, either systemically via central inhibition of FSH and boosting LH, or through paracrine actions within the ovary, remains enigmatic[6,7].

In regard to hypothalamic–pituitary function in CHA women desiring fertility, modulation of endogenous gonadotropin secretion is often achieved by clomiphene citrate or sometimes by pulsatile GnRH. Pregnancy reaching term often occurs with these regimens. But if not, gonadotropin therapy or IVF/GIFT technologies, frequently now in combination with GnRH agonists to 'down-regulate' the pituitary for prevention of LH surges, are used with significant success[8,9].

Whatever the inappropriateness of endogenous FSH/LH supply to CHA ovaries, the outcome is nearly uniform follicular atresia in high numbers at the 4–6 mm (diameter) stage. Thus, whether intrinsic to the hypothalamo–pituitary–ovarian axis, or from beyond, the milieu of CHA occurs with polycystic ovaries, usually unable to sustain follicular maturation beyond the recruitment stage. Only occasionally is a dominant follicle selected, which then proceeds to spontaneous ovulation. Interventions that succeed in fertility

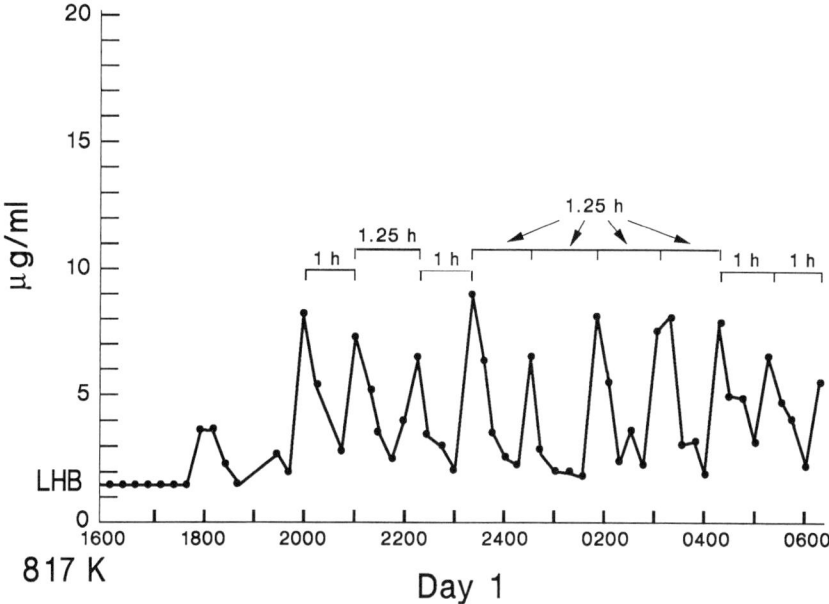

Figure 1 Pulsatile pattern of bioassayable LH in a female primate model

treatment raise the level of FSH, i.e. anti-estrogen therapy, pulsatile GnRH, FSH (or human menopausal gonadotropin) or wedge resection. We are left then to accept that ovarian function in CHA manifests a relative FSH deficiency, if not an actual diminished FSH secretion.

RECENT FINDINGS

In the experimental series that follows (Scott, R.T. *et al.*, unpublished data), it is important to notice that the GnRH antagonist subdues pituitary gonadotropin secretion almost immediately (< 24 h) after initiation of treatment; the mechanism is apparently via GnRH receptor saturation, rather than 'down-regulation', as is accomplished by GnRH agonists over about 2 weeks of treatment, i.e. paradoxical stimulation of FSH/LH secretion followed by inhibition. Projecting from the primate model, the GnRH antagonist at high doses would boldly block ovarian steroidogenesis, including chronic excessive androgen secretion. Using low doses, the pituitary would be unable to discharge an estrogen-induced preovulatory-like LH surge during gonadotropin therapy to achieve ovulation induction[10]. This approach may be useful to physicians in patient management either by simultaneous initiation of low-dose GnRH antagonist therapy in the early follicular phase, or by adding the GnRH antagonist at low doses only after gonadotropin-induced estrogen elevations threaten a potential LH surge before optimal timing of hCG injection, such as $E_2 > 250$ pg/ml.

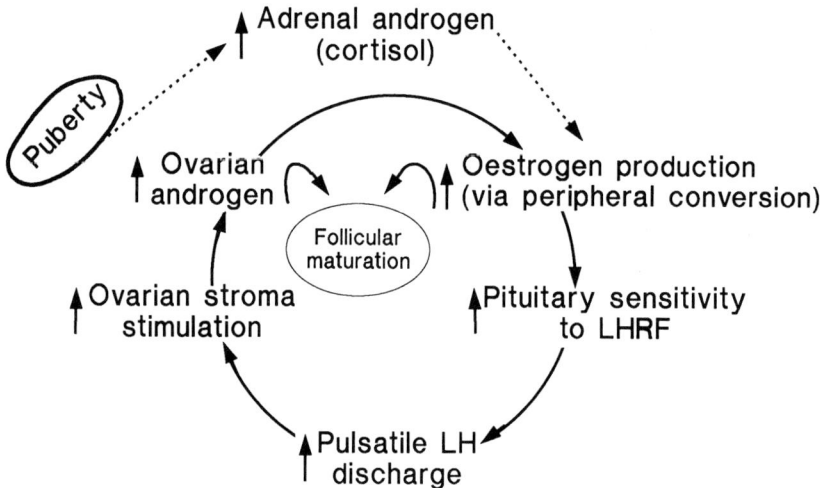

Figure 2 An exaggerated adrenarche as the pathogenesis of polycystic ovary syndrome (from Yen[5])

The primate data from our previous GnRH antagonist studies offer an additional possibility for a new therapeutic approach[11-13]. In the study below, during chronic inhibition of FSH/LH secretion by the GnRH antagonist, we could repeatedly elicit a profound and immediate LH secretory burst when i.v. boluses of GnRH were given; FSH is also transiently elevated. If these data are properly interpreted, studies may be warranted wherein patients receive GnRH antagonist and then, almost immediately, pulsatile GnRH for ovulation induction. The primate experiments below suggest these possible clinical uses of GnRH antagonists for CHA patients, as well as other indications for ovarian follicular management.

Materials and methods

Seventeen long-term ovariectomized cynomolgus monkeys (*Macaca fascicularis*) were used for this study. All primates were housed and cared for as previously described[14].

GnRH antagonist

The GnRH antagonist used in this study (ORG 30850) was provided by Organon International (Oss, Netherlands) and was dissolved in propylene glycol and water (1:1). This vehicle was also used for all control injections of monkeys. These injections were given subcutaneously.

Study design

The study was conducted in two phases. Phase 1 involved single injections of GnRH antagonist (ORG 30850) at 0.3 mg/kg (Group A, $n = 4$), 1.0 mg/kg (Group B, $n = 4$), and 3.0 mg/kg (Group C, $n = 3$). Phase 2 involved injections of the GnRH antagonist (ORG 30850) for 6 consecutive days using the same doses (Groups D to F, $n = 2$ per group). All monkeys followed the same schedule for sample collection. Daily blood samples (3.5 ml) were collected under ketamine-induced anesthesia (10 mg/kg, i.m.) for 10 days prior to GnRH antagonist administration, then daily for 22 days, and then weekly for an additional 6 weeks. An injection of vehicle (propylene glycol: water, 1:1) was given on the 3rd study day and GnRH antagonist administration was initiated on study day 10. GnRH stimulation tests (10 μg/kg, i.v.) were done on each animal the day following vehicle injection, the day following completion of GnRH antagonist administrations and weekly for 2 additional weeks. Blood samples (3 ml) were collected at -15, 0, 15, 30, 60, 90 and 120 min relative to i.v. administration of GnRH.

Hormone assays

Gonadotropin assays were performed according to previously described methodologies[15,16]. The inter- and intra-assay coefficients of variation for both LH and FSH were less than 12%.

Data analysis

For the purpose of evaluating the time required for suppression and recovery of gonadotropin concentrations from pretreatment levels, the mean baseline concentrations (days 1–10) of LH and FSH were calculated for each monkey. Monkeys were determined to be inhibited when LH and FSH concentrations fell below the 95% confidence interval of pretreatment values and to have recovered when the concentrations of LH/FSH in serum had returned to levels within these 95% confidence intervals. Due to the inconsistent nature of the FSH responsiveness during the control interval, only LH responsiveness to exogenous GnRH administration was examined statistically. LH concentrations on days of GnRH tests were normalized with respect to baseline by subtracting the mean LH concentrations of the -15 and 0 min samples from all subsequent determinations for the next 2 h. The parameters analyzed were maximum GnRH-induced LH pulse amplitude (Δ_{max}), time of maximum amplitude (t_{max}) and area under the GnRH-induced LH curve (AUC) from zero time until the final challenge test specimen was drawn at $+120$ min.

Results

In most monkeys LH and FSH inhibition was achieved by 24 h (Table 2). In one case (K5, Group E), FSH levels were very low throughout so that FSH suppression could not be measured. For monkey K2 (Group B), FSH levels were not inhibited until day 2. Long-term inhibition of gonadotropin concentrations (> 2 weeks) was achieved in all monkeys receiving a cumulative dose of at least 1 mg/kg. However, two of the four females receiving a single injection of 0.3 mg/kg also exhibited long-term effects. Of the remaining

Table 2 Pattern of gonadotropin secretory inhibition and recovery in ovariectomized monkeys given GnRH antagonist ORG 30850

Group	Treatment (mg/kg)	Monkey	Day of 1st inhibition LH	Day of 1st inhibition FSH	Day of recovery LH	Day of recovery FSH
A	0.3	P19	1	1	6	3
		P2	1	1	36	> 64
		L4	1	1	13	6
		P13	1	1	29	> 64
B	1.0	K2	1	2	29	29
		P20	1	1	> 64	> 64
		P21	1	1	18	16
		T5	1	1	28	18
C	3.0	67A	1	1	35	> 63
		906N	1	1	42	> 63
		C45	1	1	28	> 63
D	0.3	J2	1	1	20	16
		39	1	1	35	38
E	1.0 × 6	K5	1	none*	36	none*
		K12X	1	1	> 36	> 36
F	3.0 × 6	C15B	1	1	> 63	> 63
		L16	1	1	> 64	> 64

* Very low FSH levels throughout

two monkeys, one (P19) was inhibited for less than 1 week, the other (L4) for 1–2 weeks (Table 2).

Pituitary responsiveness to serial GnRH i.v. challenge tests was retained throughout the study. Immediately (1 day) following ORG 30850-induced gonadotropin inhibition, pituitary responsiveness was enhanced. LH concentrations reached higher peak amplitudes (Table 3), peaked more rapidly (15–30 min vs. 90 or 120 min) (Table 4) and sustained the release of more LH (Table 5). This striking enhancement of LH secretory responsiveness decreased with time after antagonist administration, returning to a pretreatment pattern of responsiveness approximately coincident with the ultimate recovery of tonic gonadotropin concentrations.

Discussion

These results demonstrate that ORG 30850 is capable of inducing long-term inhibition of gonadotropin concentrations in ovariectomized cynomolgus monkeys in a very similar fashion to that already observed for Antide (Nal-Lys)[13,17,18]. It is implied from the data, though not yet proven, that the long-term effects of ORG 30850 on gonadotropin levels are due to a prolonged presence of ORG 30850 in the peripheral circulation, perhaps via significant binding to serum proteins with dissociation rates sufficient to maintain lengthy intervals of pituitary gonadotropin secretory inhibition[18]. The mechanisms whereby pituitary responsiveness to exogenously adminis-

Table 3 Maximum i.v. GnRH-induced LH secretory amplitude (Δ_{max}) in ovariectomized monkeys given GnRH antagonist ORG 30850. Superscript numbers indicate ranking within individual primate responses

Group	Treatment (mg/kg)	Monkey	Control −6	1	6	13	20
					Days relative to GnRH antagonist treatment		
A	0.3	P19	171[5]	274[2]	309[1]	269[3]	186[4]
		P2	182[4]	336[2]	713[1]	327[3]	172[5]
		L4	274[3]	319[2]	331[1]	51[5]	80[4]
		P13	270[3]	394[1]	377[2]	208[4]	140[5]
B	1.0	K2	93[5]	109[4]	268[1]	251[2]	140[3]
		P20	369[3]	375[2]	399[1]	302[4]	182[5]
		P21	196[4]	350[2]	544[1]	248[3]	147[5]
		T5	166[4]	333[2]	488[1]	177[3]	127[5]
C	3.0	67A	518[3]	473[4]	888[1]	644[2]	309[5]
		906N	112[5]	224[3]	348[1]	268[2]	175[4]
		C45	394[5]	620[2]	1039[1]	528[3]	469[4]
D	0.3 × 6	J2	52[3]	—	98[2]	131[1]	23[4]
		39	284[3]	—	622[1]	594[2]	104[4]
E	1.0 × 6	K5	222[4]	—	305[1]	268[3]	304[2]
		K12X	105[1]	—	85[2]	25[3]	7[4]
F	3.0 × 6	C15B	337[3]	—	647[1]	556[2]	325[4]
		L16	339[3]	—	784[1]	519[2]	278[4]

Table 4 Time of maximum i.v. GnRH-induced LH pulse amplitude (t_{max}) in ovariectomized monkeys receiving GnRH antagonist ORG 30850

Group	Treatment (mg/kg)	Monkey	Control −6	1	6	13	20
					Days relative to GnRH antagonist treatment		
A	0.3	P19	60	30	60	60	30
		P2	90	15	30	15	30
		L4	90	30	15	120	60
		P13	120	15	30	60	30
B	1.0	K2	90	30	15	30	15
		P20	90	30	30	15	60
		P21	60	15	30	15	90
		T5	60	15	30	15	90
C	3.0	67A	120	30	15	15	15
		906N	120	30	15	15	15
		C45	90	30	15	15	30
D	0.3 × 6	J2	120	—	30	30	90
		39	120	—	15	15	90
E	1.0 × 6	K5	90	—	15	15	15
		K12X	120	—	15	15	15
F	3.0 × 6	C15B	120	—	15	15	15
		L16	60	—	15	15	15

Table 5 Total i.v. GnRH-induced LH release (AUC) over 2 h in ovariectomized monkeys given GnRH antagonist ORG 30850. Superscript numbers indicate ranking within individual primate responses

			Days relative to GnRH antagonist treatment				
	Treatment		Control				
Group	(mg/kg)	Monkey	−6	1	6	13	20
A	0.3	P19	15180^5	19425^2	26333^1	18060^3	16845^4
		P2	17580^4	29055^2	51038^1	24593^3	14355^5
		L4	22493^3	23183^2	29228^1	4943^5	7163^4
		P13	19755^4	23520^2	32723^1	20190^3	13065^5
B	1.0	K2	9015^3	8468^4	19343^1	16433^2	8018^5
		P20	34958^1	26453^3	30203^2	23820^4	14183^5
		P21	13883^4	20640^2	34710^1	15203^3	11535^5
		T5	14685^4	23423^2	38985^3	16530^3	11978^5
C	3.0	67A	35843^4	36863^3	68955^1	46373^2	25200^5
		906N	10553^4	19230^2	27510^1	16695^3	10373^5
		C45	35715^4	49440^2	78233^1	41243^3	35205^5
D	0.3 × 6	J2	2805^3	—	8145^2	13988^1	1950^4
		39	19920^3	—	39143^2	39690^1	10223^4
E	1.0 × 6	K5	20925^1	—	18338^3	13485^4	18413^2
		K12X	8730^1	—	5873^2	1515^3	323^4
F	3.0 × 6	C15B	22830^3	—	37568^1	24068^2	15105^4
		L16	26415^2	—	43733^1	24608^3	13883^4

tered GnRH is enhanced remain enigmatic; however, we favor an interpretation that there is a requirement for a threshold concentration of GnRH before sufficient displacement of GnRH antagonist from the GnRH receptors, thereby eliciting an LH secretory response. Another possibility is that, although endogenous release of gonadotropins is blocked by GnRH antagonist administration, perhaps synthesis continues for at least part of the time, leading to an increase in intracellular LH storage. This mechanism may be reflected in the earlier and greater amounts of LH released via the GnRH i.v. bolus.

Retention of pituitary responsiveness to exogenously administered GnRH, in the face of chronic GnRH antagonist-induced inhibition of endogenous gonadotropin release, may be clinically useful. Theoretically, in conditions such as chronic hyperandrogenic amenorrhea, ovulation induction may be improved either by administering human menopausal gonadotropins or pulsatile GnRH at a dose and frequency compatible with physiological ovarian functions.

REFERENCES

1. Goldzieher, J.W. and Axelrod, L.R. (1963). Clinical and biochemical features of polycystic ovarian disease. *Fertil. Steril.*, **14**, 631–53
2. Judd, H.L. (1978). Endocrinology of polycystic ovarian disease. *Clin. Obstet. Gynecol.*, **21**, 99–114

3. Yen, S.S.C. (1980). The polycystic ovary syndrome. *Clin. Endocrinol.*, **12**, 177–208
4. Franks, S. (1989). Polycystic ovary syndrome: a changing perspective. *Clin. Endocrinol.*, **31**, 87–120
5. Yen, S.S.C. (1986). Chronic anovulation caused by peripheral endocrine disorders. In Yen, S.S.C. and Jaffe, R.B. (eds.) *Reproductive Endocrinology*, pp. 441–99. (Philadelphia: W.B. Saunders)
6. Tanabe, K., Gagliano, P., Channing, C.P., Nakamura, Y., Yoshimura, Y., Iizuka, R., Fortuny, A., Sulewski, J. and Rezai, N. (1983). Levels of inhibin-F activity and steroids in human follicular fluid from normal women and women with polycystic ovarian disease. *J. Clin. Endocrinol. Metab.*, **57**, 24–31
7. Buckler, H.M., McLachlan, R.I., MacLachlan, V.B., Healy, D.L. and Burger, H.G. (1988). Serum inhibin levels in polycystic ovary syndrome: basal levels and response to luteinizing hormone-releasing hormone agonist and exogenous gonadotropin administration. *J. Clin. Endocrinol. Metab.*, **66**, 798–803
8. Meldrum, D.R., Wisot, A., Hamilton, F., Gutley, A.L., Kempton, W. and Huyhn, D. (1989). Routine pituitary suppression with leuprolide before ovarian stimulation for oocyte retrieval. *Fertil. Steril.*, **51**, 455–9
9. Droesch, K., Muasher, S.J., Brzyski, R.G., Jones, G.S., Simonetti, S., Liu, H.-C. and Rosenwaks, Z. (1989). Value of suppression with a gonadotropin-releasing hormone agonist prior to gonadotropin stimulation for *in vitro* fertilization. *Fertil. Steril.*, **51**, 292–7
10. Kenigsberg, D., Littman, B.A. and Hodgen, G.D. (1984). Medical hypophysectomy. I. Dose-response using a gonadotropin-releasing hormone antagonist. *Fertil. Steril.*, **42**, 112–15
11. Kenigsberg, D. and Hodgen, G.D. (1986). Ovulation inhibition by administration of weekly gonadotropin-releasing hormone antagonist. *J. Clin. Endocrinol. Metab.*, **62**, 734–8
12. Chillik, C.F., Itskovitz, J., Hahn, D.W., McGuire, J.L., Danforth, D.R. and Hodgen, G.D. (1987). Characterizing pituitary response to a gonadotropin-releasing hormone (GnRH) antagonist in monkeys: tonic follicle-stimulating hormone/luteinizing hormone secretion versus acute GnRH challenge tests before, during and after treatment. *Fertil. Steril.*, **48**, 480–5
13. Leal, J.A., Gordon, K., Williams, R.F., Danforth, D.R., Roh, S.I. and Hodgen, G.D. (1989). Probing studies on multiple dose effects of Antide (Nal-Lys) GnRH antagonist in ovariectomized monkeys. *Contraception*, **40**, 623–33
14. Goodman, A.L., Descalzi, C.D., Johnson, D.K. and Hodgen, G.D. (1977). Composite patterns of circulating LH, FSH, estradiol and progesterone during the menstrual cycle in cynomolgus monkeys. *Proc. Soc. Exp. Biol. Med.*, **155**, 479–81
15. Goodman, A.L., Nixon, W.E., Johnson, D.K. and Hodgen, G.D. (1977). Regulation of folliculogenesis in the cycling rhesus monkey: selection of the dominant follicle. *Endocrinology*, **100**, 155–61
16. Hodgen, G.D., Tullner, W.W., Vaitukaitis, J.L., Ward, D.N. and Ross, G.T. (1974). Specific radioimmunoassay of chorionic gonadotropins during implantation in rhesus monkeys. *J. Clin. Endocrinol. Metab.*, **39**, 457–64
17. Leal, J.A., Williams, R.F., Danforth, D.R., Gordon, K. and Hodgen, G.D. (1988). Prolonged duration of gonadotropin inhibition by a third generation GnRH antagonist. *J. Clin. Endocrinol. Metab.*, **67**, 1325–7
18. Danforth, D.R., Gordon, K., Leal, J.A., Williams, R.F. and Hodgen, G.D. (1990). Extended presence of Antide (Nal-Lys GnRH antagonist) in circulation: prolonged duration of gonadotropin inhibition may derive from Antide binding to serum proteins. *J. Clin. Endocrinol. Metab.*, **70**, 554–6

5

Adrenal androgens and chronic anovulation

M.I. New, M. Zerah and C. Crawford

STEROID 21-HYDROXYLASE

Deficiency of the enzyme steroid 21-hydroxylase, required for synthesis of the essential adrenal hormones cortisol and aldosterone, is the most commonly occurring error in steroidogenesis[1]. Classical genetic studies showed linkage of this deficiency with HLA (the human major histocompatibility complex) on the short arm of chromosome 6[2,3] and the molecular genetics of the steroid 21-hydroxylase enzyme of the adrenal cortex continue to be intensively researched[4].

Clinical consequences arise primarily from accumulation of cortisol precursors proximal to the impaired 21-hydroxylating step and the shunting of these steroid prehormones into androgen synthetic pathways. Severe deficiencies of 21-hydroxylase are the basis of 95% of cases of the classical disorder, congenital adrenal hyperplasia (CAH). Milder adrenal 21-hydroxylase defects, termed non-classical, are more widely expressed and are often the basis of more generalized androgen excess states.

In the classical deficiency, prenatal elevations of adrenal androgens cause ambiguous genitalia in affected females, and in 75% of cases impaired synthesis of the mineralocorticoid aldosterone results in inability to retain serum sodium ('salt wasting') with acidosis, hypovolemia and shock. Postnatally, both sexes manifest rapid somatic growth with accelerated skeletal maturation, early closure of the epiphyses, and short adult stature. Other symptoms of androgen excess include abnormal patterns of body hair and decreased fertility.

STEROID 11β-HYDROXYLASE AND 3β-HYDROXYSTEROID DEHYDROGENASE

Steroid 11β-hydroxylase

Defects in steroid 11β-hydroxylase activity account for approximately 5% of all cases of CAH. This enzyme deficiency results in a rise of 11-

deoxysteroids and metabolites. The index serum compounds are 11-deoxycortisol (compound S) and 11-deoxycorticosterone. 11-Deoxycorticosterone itself is a moderately potent salt-retaining steroid and elevated 11-deoxycorticosterone causes sodium retention, plasma volume expansion and suppression of plasma renin activity. Hypokalemia and alkalosis resulting from mineralocorticoid hormone excess are inconstant features of this form of congenital adrenal hyperplasia.

Androgen excess results from cortisol precursor accumulation in 11β-hydroxylase as in 21-hydroxylase deficiency. As in 21-hydroxylase deficiency, excess fetal androgen production causes prenatal virilization of females, resulting in ambiguous external genitalia with normal female internal reproductive organs. In newborn males with 11β-hydroxylase deficiency, the external genitalia may be normal, but in either sex virilization ensues postnatally if the disorder is untreated. Hypertension allows clinical distinction of these two virilizing forms of congenital adrenal hyperplasia.

Steroid 11β-hydroxylase deficiency is transmitted as an autosomal recessive (as for all the adrenal steroidogenic enzymes). The gene for the steroid 11β-hydroxylase enzyme has been assigned to human chromosome 8[5].

3β-Hydroxysteroid dehydrogenase deficiency

Deficiency of 3β-hydroxysteroid (3β-ol) dehydrogenase affects the synthesis of all classes of adrenocortical steroids and produces elevated serum levels of Δ^5-steroids pregnenolone, 17α-hydroxypregnenolone and dehydroepiandrosterone. Unlike steroid 21-hydroxylase, the 3β-ol dehydrogenase enzyme (3β-HSD) is active in the gonads as well as in the adrenal. Androgen deficiency resulting from the enzymatic defect of 3β-HSD may cause ambiguous genitalia in genetic male newborns. Clitoral enlargement in some affected females is due to the very high levels of the weakly androgenic dehydroepiandrosterone undergoing peripheral conversion to more potent androgens. Aldosterone deficiency in classical cases of 3β-HSD results in salt wasting, while in several cases the ability to conserve sodium has been intact.

CLASSICAL AND NON-CLASSICAL FORMS OF THE ADRENAL ENZYME DEFECTS

Partial enzyme blocks of adrenal steroid production are more common. Patients with these non-classical forms are born without symptoms of adrenal disease but may develop signs of androgen excess later in life. A subset of non-classical 21-hydroxylase deficiency individuals are overtly asymptomatic when detected (usually as part of a family study), but longitudinal follow-up of such patients has shown hyperandrogenic symptoms to wax and wane with time[6,7].

Classical 21-hydroxylase deficiency is found in about 1 in 12 500 births[1]. Non-classical 21-hydroxylase deficiency is far more frequent, occurring in up to 3% of certain ethnic groups. This figure, derived from combined analysis of hormonal data and HLA associations in parents of patients with 21-hydroxylase deficiency, indicates that non-classical 21-hydroxylase deficiency is the most common autosomal recessive disorder in man.

While 11β-hydroxylase deficiency accounts for approximately 5% of the worldwide cases of congenital adrenal hyperplasia, in Israel it has been found that 20% of that country's population with congenital adrenal hyperplasia was comprised of 11β-hydroxylase deficiency patients[8] (1 per 60 000 live births). This unusual incidence stemmed from Israeli families of North African origin, particularly from Morocco and Tunisia. Turkish Jews also have been found to carry the 11β-hydroxylase deficiency gene in high frequency[9,10].

Although it has been claimed that late-onset 3β-HSD deficiency is the second most common steroidogenic defect[11], no epidemiological studies to date have verified the true frequency. There have been no reports of geographic clusters of 3β-HSD deficiency, nor is there a recognized ethnic predominance.

NON-CLASSICAL 21-HYDROXYLASE DEFICIENCY

Diagnosis of a 21-hydroxylase defect by serum assay was made possible in the early 1970s with the availability of a radioimmunoassay for 17-hydroxyprogesterone[12-14]. The HLA associations for non-classical 21-hydroxylase deficiency[15] are distinct from those found in classical 21-hydroxylase deficiency and are ethnic group-specific[16,17].

Clinical symptomatology of non-classical 21-hydroxylase deficiency is variable, and may present at any age. Non-classical 21-hydroxylase deficiency can result in premature development of pubic hair in children[18], and early fusion of epiphyseal growth plates with short stature[19].

Severe cystic acne refractory to oral antibiotics and retinoic acid has been attributed to non-classical 21-hydroxylase deficiency[20].

Additionally, male-pattern baldness in young women may be the sole presenting symptom. Menarche may occur prematurely or may be delayed and the expression of ovarian function varies from oligomenorrhea and amenorrhea to regular cyclic menses. Infertility is reported in untreated male and female patients[21-23].

Retrospective analysis of women presenting to this institution for hirsutism and oligomenorrhea revealed non-classical 21-hydroxylase deficiency in 16 of 108 (14%)[24]. In other published series this prevalence ranges from 1.2% to 30%[25-28]. A total of 15% met the hormonal criteria for the diagnosis of mild 3β-HSD deficiency[29-31]. The disparity in frequency of non-classical 21-hydroxylase deficiency in different reports may be attributed to differences in the ethnic groups studied.

Evaluation of data gathered in our clinic on 48 women with non-classical 21-hydroxylase deficiency indicates that hirsutism occurs in 83% of cases, irregular menses in 52%, acne in 19%, clitoromegaly in 11%, obesity in 8% and hair loss in 3%; in 11% of the patients premature menarche is also found. However, symptoms of androgen excess could not be identified in

8% of our non-classical 21-hydroxylase deficiency patients diagnosed during the course of family studies. Infertility may be the only presenting complaint in women with the disease. Our unpublished study reveals that 16% (or 4 out of 25) of infertile women are affected.

Although the androgen profile in serum and urine in both the basal and adrenocorticotropic hormone (ACTH)-stimulated states may not be markedly different from that of women with polycystic ovary syndrome, the 17-hydroxyprogesterone response to ACTH clearly differentiates the patients with an adrenal 21-hydroxylase defect[24]. ACTH tests are required for the differential diagnosis. Sonograms of the ovary do not distinguish women with excess androgens due to polycystic ovary syndrome from those with non-classical 21-hydroxylase deficiency. Similarly, ACTH tests are necessary to differentiate polycystic ovary syndrome from non-classical 21-hydroxylase deficiency after luteinizing hormone releasing hormone (LHRH) testing of pituitary gonadotropin secretion. The response to LHRH is variably abnormal in virilized women with non-classical 21-hydroxylase deficiency[32,33].

Treatment with glucocorticoids suppresses adrenal androgen overproduction, and with time, clinical signs of androgen excess show improvement. Given the 9-month life expectancy of established hair follicles, remission of hirsutism generally takes at least 1–2 years. Reversal of infertility in women has been noted folowing glucocorticoid therapy[22,34–37]. One study[38] reported that five patients with postmenarchal onset of 21-hydroxylase deficiency resumed regular menses and demonstrated adequate suppression of 17-ketosteroids and pregnanetriol within 2 months after beginning glucocorticoid therapy alone. Another study[23] found that of 18 infertile women with acne and/or facial hirsutism and hormonal criteria consistent with 21-hydroxylase deficiency, five conceived after 2–7 months of prednisone treatment alone. Four more women conceived within 2 months of the addition of clomiphene to the therapeutic regimen. Hormonal profiles after initiation of therapy were not reported in this study. In a recent review of patients in our clinic, two of three infertile non-classical 21-hydroxylase deficiency women became pregnant after $1–1\frac{1}{2}$ years of glucocorticoid therapy.

Hormonal standards for genotyping 21-hydroxylase deficiency

In our experience the best test for genotyping for 21-hydroxylase deficiency has proven to be an ACTH stimulation test measuring the serum concentration of 17-hydroxyprogesterone at 0 and 60 min after intravenous bolus administration of 0.25 mg Cortrosyn (synthetic $ACTH_{1-24}$)[39]. The hormonal responses of classically affected, non-classically affected, heterozygote (carrier), and genetically unaffected subjects form a regression line on a standard x, y plot[39]. Reference to this graph permits assignment of the test subject to one of these defined groups and thus determination of the 21-hydroxylase genotype. Due to diurnal variation of 17-hydroxyprogesterone, the baseline serum or salivary[40] concentration of 17-hydroxyprogesterone in the early morning (before 8:00 a.m.) may be useful as a screening test for 21-hydroxylase deficiency, but later discussion[31,41] has supported the original observation that ACTH stimulation testing is the most definitive diagnostic test[39].

NON-CLASSICAL 11β-HYDROXYLASE DEFICIENCY

As in 21-hydroxylase deficiency, there is a wide range of clinical expression of non-classical 11β-hydroxylase deficiency[42]. Mild, late-onset, and even cryptic forms of 11β-hydroxylase deficiency have been reported[42–47] and may represent allelic variants.

NON-CLASSICAL 3β-HYDROXYSTEROID DEHYDROGENASE DEFICIENCY

Non-classical 3β-HSD deficiency is usually identified in girls with premature adrenarche or in adolescent or young adult women with hirsutism and oligomenorrhea[48]. ACTH-stimulated adrenal hormone profiles allowed differentiation of this subgroup from women classified as having polycystic ovarian syndrome[24]. Relatively little is known about non-classical 3β-HSD in males.

In a study of hirsute pubertal and postpubertal women undergoing ACTH stimulation testing in this clinic[24], post-ACTH 17α-hydroxypregnenolone (Δ^5-17P) and dehydroepiandrosterone levels in 17 of 116 hirsute women were more than 2 standard deviations above the mean for non-hirsute women and completely outside the normal range. This hormonal response was taken to establish mild 3β-HSD deficiency. The 17α-hydroxypregnenolone and dehydroepiandrosterone levels in these women were significantly ($p < 0.05$) higher than those of hirsute women with non-classical 21-hydroxylase deficiency, although some values overlapped between the two groups. ACTH-stimulated 17-hydroxyprogesterone and cortisol levels in these hirsute women did not significantly differ from the same ACTH-stimulated levels in normal women. The ratios of ACTH-stimulated 17α-hydroxypregnenolone/17-hydroxyprogesterone and 17α-hydroxypregnenolone/cortisol in the 17 hirsute women were more than 2 standard deviations above the normal mean.

Short adult height is also common with 3β-HSD deficiency. Seven of 17 women have reported final heights at least 5–12 cm below their parents' heights. Premature pubarche was found in five out of 11 women with non-classical 3β-HSD. Of note is the fact that two women who did not have menstrual abnormalities had polycystic changes of the ovaries on pelvic ultrasonogram.

Random serum LH concentrations in four of the 17 women were elevated ($> 29\,mIU/ml$). These four women had menstrual abnormalities; of these four, three underwent pelvic sonography, with normal findings in one and abnormal findings in two. Serum prolactin levels in 16 women measured were in the normal range (4–22 ng/ml (normal range, $< 25\,ng/ml$)).

Four of the 17 women underwent adrenal computer assisted tomography, which showed adrenal hyperplasia. One of the 17 women had abdominal ultrasonographic studies, which revealed enlargement of the left adrenal, while the right adrenal was not visualized[24]. These data indicate that ACTH testing is required for polycystic ovary syndrome with no adrenal steroidogenic defect to be distinguished from non-classical 3β-HSD with ovarian involvement.

CONCLUSION

The syndrome of polycystic ovaries includes a subgroup of women with non-classical 21-hydroxylase deficiency, non-classical 3β-hydroxysteroid dehydrogenase deficiency, non-classical 11β-hydroxylase deficiency and hyperandrogenism caused by these adrenal steroidogenic defects, which are easily treated by low-dose glucocorticoids. Identification of these disorders via ACTH testing is cost-effective in patients with symptoms of androgen excess as well as in patients with reduced fertility and asymptomatic family members of patients with proven adrenal steroidogenic defects.

ACKNOWLEDGEMENTS

Studies described in this article have been supported by US Public Health Service grant HD00072 and General Clinical Research Centers grant RR47 of the National Institutes of Health (NIH). Current support from the Kalikow Foundation is also acknowledged.

REFERENCES

1. New, M.I., White, P.C., Pang, S., Dupont, B. and Speiser, P.W. (1989). The adrenal hyperplasias. In Scriver, C.L., Beaudet, A.L., Sly, W.S. and Valle, D. (eds.) *The Metabolic Basis of Inherited Disease*, 6th edn., pp. 1881–917. (New York: McGraw-Hill)
2. Dupont, B., Oberfield, S.E., Smithwick, E.M. *et al.* (1977). Close genetic linkage between HLA and congenital adrenal hyperplasia (21-hydroxylase deficiency). *Lancet*, 2, 1309
3. Levine, L.S., Zachmann, M., New, M.I., Prader, A., Pollack, M.S., O'Neill, G.J., Yang, S.Y., Oberfield, S.E. and Dupont, B. (1978). Genetic mapping of the 21-hydroxylase deficiency gene within the HLA linkage group. *N. Engl. J. Med.*, **299**, 911–15
4. White, P.C., New, M.I. and Dupont, B. (1987). Congenital adrenal hyperplasia. *N. Engl. J. Med.*, **316**, 1519–24 and 1580–6
5. Chua, S.C., Szabo, P., Vitek, A., Grzeschik, K.-H., John, M. and White, P.C. (1987). Cloning of cDNA encoding steroid 11β-hydroxylase (p450c11). *Proc. Natl. Acad. Sci. USA*, **84**, 7193–7
6. Faglia, G., Travaglini, P., Neri, V., Farrari, C., Gattinoni, L. and Acerbi, L. (1969). Occurrence of a virilizing syndrome with 21-hydroxylase deficiency after pregnancy. *J. Clin. Endocrinol. Metab.*, **29**, 1325–9
7. Leichter, S.B. and Jacobs, L.S. (1976). Normal gestation and diminished androgen responsiveness in an untreated patient with 21-hydroxylase deficiency. *J. Clin. Endocrinol. Metab.*, **42**, 575–82
8. Porter, B., Finzi, M., Leiberman, E. and Moses, S. (1977). The syndrome of congenital adrenal hyperplasia in Israel. *Pediatrician*, **6**, 100–5
9. Blunck, W. and Bierich, J.R. (1968). CAH with 11β-hydroxylase deficiency. A case report and contribution to diagnosis. *Acta Paediatr. Scand.*, **57**, 157–61

10. Zachmann, M., Tassinari, D. and Prader, A. (1983). Clinical and biochemical variability of congenital adrenal hyperplasia due to 11β-OHD. A study of 25 patients. *J. Clin. Endocrinol. Metab.*, **56**, 222–9

11. Bongiovanni, A.M. (1986). Late-onset adrenal hyperplasia (letter). *N. Engl. J. Med.*, **314**, 450

12. Abraham, G.E., Swerdloff, R.S., Tulchinsky, D., Hopper, K. and Odell, W.D. (1971). Radioimmunoassay of plasma 17-hydroxyprogesterone. *J. Clin. Endocrinol. Metab.*, **33**, 42–6

13. Blankstein, J., Faiman, C., Reyes, F.I., Schroeder, M.L. and Winter, J.S.D. (1980). Adult-onset familial adrenal 21-hydroxylase deficiency. *Am. J. Med.*, **68**, 441

14. Migeon, C.J., Rosenwaks, Z., Lee, P.A., Urban, M.D. and Bias, W.B. (1980). The attenuated form of congenital adrenal hyperplasia as an allelic form of 21-hydroxylase deficiency. *J. Clin. Endocrinol. Metab.*, **51**, 647

15. Pollack, M.S., Levine, L.S., O'Neill, G.J., Pang, S., Lorenzen, F., Kohn, B., Rondanini, G.F., Chiumello, G., New, M.I. and Dupont, B. (1981). HLA linkage and B14,DR1,Bfs haplotype association with the genes for late onset and cryptic 21-hydroxylase deficiency. *Am. J. Hum. Genet.*, **33**, 540–50

16. Laron, Z., Pollack, M.S., Zamir, R., Roitman, A., Dickerman, Z., Levine, L.S., Lorenzen, F., O'Neill, G.J., Pang, S., New, M.I. and Dupont, B. (1980). Late onset 21-hydroxylase deficiency and HLA in the Ashkenazi population; a new allele at the 21-hydroxylase locus. *Hum. Immunol.*, **1**, 55–66

17. Speiser, P.W., Dupont, B., Rubinstein, P., Piazza, A., Kastelan, A. and New, M.I. (1985). High frequency of nonclassical steroid 21-hydroxylase deficiency. *Am. J. Hum. Genet.*, **37**, 650–67

18. Kohn, B., Levine, L.S., Pollack, M.S., Pang, S., Lorenzen, F., Levy, D., Lerner, A., Rondanini, G.F., Dupont, B. and New, M.I. (1982). Late-onset steroid 21-hydroxylase deficiency: a variant of classical congenital adrenal hyperplasia. *J. Clin. Endocrinol. Metab.*, **55**, 817–27

19. New, M.I., Gertner, J.M., Speiser, P.W. and del Balzo, P. (1988). Growth and final height in classical and nonclassical 21-hydroxylase deficiency. *Acta Paediatr. Jpn.*, **30** (Suppl.), 79–88

20. Rose, L.I., Newmark, S.R., Strauss, J.S. and Pochi, P.E. (1976). Adrenocortical hydroxylase deficiencies in acne vulgaris. *J. Invest. Dermatol.*, **66**, 324–6

21. Mahesh, V., Greenblatt, R. and Coniff, R. (1968). Adrenal hyperplasia – a case report of delayed onset of the congenital form or an acquired form. *J. Clin. Endocrinol. Metab.*, **28**, 619–23

22. Sarris, S., Dwyer, G., Ward, R., Lawrence, D., McGarrigle, H. and Little, V. (1978). The treatment of mild adrenal hyperplasia and associated infertility with prednisone. *J. Obstet. Gynecol.*, **85**, 251–3

23. Birnbaum, M.D. and Rose, L.I. (1979). The partial adrenocortical hydroxylase deficiency syndrome in infertile women. *Fertil. Steril.*, **32**, 536–41

24. Pang, S., Lerner, A., Stoner, E., Levine, L., Oberfield, S., Engle, I. and New. M.I. (1985). Late-onset steroid 3β-hydroxysteroid dehydrogenase deficiency. I. A cause of hirsutism in pubertal and postpubertal women. *J. Clin. Endocrinol. Metab.*, **60**, 428–36

25. Child, D.F., Bullock, D.E. and Anderson, D.E. (1980). Adrenal steroidogenesis in hirsute women. *Clin. Endocrinol. (Oxf.)*, **12**, 595–601

26. Gibson, M., Lackritz, R., Schiff, I. and Tulchinsky, D. (1980). Abnormal adrenal responses to adrenocorticotropic hormone in hyperandrogenic women. *Fertil. Steril.*, **33**, 43–8

27. Lobo, R.A. and Goebelsmann, U. (1980). Adult manifestation of congenital adrenal hyperplasia due to incomplete 21-hydroxylase deficiency mimicking polycystic ovarian disease. *Am. J. Obstet. Gynecol.*, **138**, 720–6

28. Chrousos, G.P., Loriaux, D.L., Mann, D.L. and Cutler, G.B. (1982). Late-onset 21-hydroxylase deficiency mimicking idiopathic hirsutism or polycystic ovarian disease. An allelic variant of congenital virilizing adrenal hyperplasia with a milder enzymatic defect. *Ann. Intern. Med.*, **96**, 143–8

29. Chrousos, G.P., Loriaux, D.L., Mann, D. and Cutler, G.B. (1982). Late onset 21-hydroxylase deficiency is an allelic variant of congenital adrenal hyperplasia characterized by attenuated clinical expression and different HLA haplotype association. *Horm. Res.*, **16**, 193–200

30. Chetkowski, R., DeFazio, J., Shamonki, I., Judd, H.L. and Chang, R.J. (1984). The incidence

of late-onset congenital andrenal hyperplasia due to 21-hydroxylase deficiency among hirsute women. *J. Clin. Endocrinol. Metab.*, **58**, 595–8

31. Kuttenn, F., Couillin, P., Girard, F., Billaud, L., Vincens, M., Boucekkine, C., Thalabard, J-C., Maudelonde, T., Spritzer, P., Mowszowicz, I., Boue, A. and Mauvais-Jarvis, P. (1986). Late-onset adrenal hyperplasia in hirsutism. *N. Engl. J. Med.*, **313**, 224–31

32. Gangemi, M., Benato, M., Guacci, A.M. and Menghetti, G. (1983). Stimulation tests in adrenogenital syndrome induced by 21-hydroxylase deficit. *Clin. Expr. Obstet. Gynecol.*, **10**, 127

33. Speiser, P.W., Drucker, S. and New, M.I. (1987). Hypothalamic–pituitary–gonadal axis in nonclassical 21-hydroxylase deficiency. Program and Abstracts, 69th Annual Meeting of the Endocrine Society, Indianapolis, Indiana, June 1987. *Endocrinology*, **120** (Suppl.), 171/A602

34. Jones, H.W. and Jones, G.E.S. (1954). The gynecological aspects of adrenal hyperplasia and allied disorders. *Am. J. Obstet. Gynecol.*, **68**, 1330–65

35. Decourt, M.J., Jayle, M.F. and Baulieu, E. (1957). Virilisme cliniquement tardif avec excretion de pregnanetriol et insuffisance de la production du cortisol. *Ann. Endocrinol. (Paris)*, **18**, 416

36. Wilson, R. and Keating, F. (1958). Pregnancy following treatment of CAH with cortisone. *Am. J. Obstet. Gynecol.*, **76**, 388–97

37. Jefferies, W.M., Wier, W.C., Weir, D.R. and Prouty, R.L. (1958). The use of cortisone and related steroids in infertility. *Fertil. Steril.*, **9**, 145–7

38. Riddick, D.H. and Hammond, C.B. (1975). Adrenal virilism due to 21-hydroxylase deficiency in the postmenarchial female. *Obstet. Gynecol.*, **45**, 21–4

39. New, M.I., Lorenzen, F., Lerner, A.J., Kohn, B., Oberfield, S.E., Pollack, M.S., Dupont, B., Stoner, E., Levy, D.J., Pang, S. and Levine, L.S. (1983). Genotyping steroid 21-hydroxylase deficiency: hormonal reference data. *J. Clin. Endocrinol. Metab.*, **57**,320–6

40. Zerah, M., Pang, S. and New, M.I. (1987). Morning salivary 17-hydroxyprogesterone is a useful screening test for nonclassical 21-hydroxylase deficiency. *J. Clin. Endocrinol. Metab.*, **65**, 227–32

41. Kuttenn, F. (1986). Late-onset adrenal hyperplasia (response to letters). *N. Engl. J. Med.*, **314**, 450–1

42. Rosler, A. and Leiberman, E. (1984). Enzymatic defects of steroidogenesis: 11β-hydroxylase deficiency congenital adrenal hyperplasia. In New, M.I. and Levine, L.S. (eds.) *Adrenal Diseases in Childhood*, (*Pediatr. Adolesc. Endocrinol.*, Vol. 13), pp.47–71. (Basel: S. Karger)

43. Gabrilove, J.L., Sharma, D.C. and Dorfman, R.I. (1965). Adrenocortical 11β-hydroxylase deficiency and virilism first manifest in the adult woman. *N. Engl. J. Med.*, **272**, 1189–94

44. Newmark, S., Dluhy, R.G., Williams, G.H., Pochi, P. and Rose, L.I. (1977). Partial 11- and 21-hydroxylase deficiencies in hirsute women. *Am. J. Obstet. Gynecol.*, **127**, 594–8

45. Cathelineau, G., Brerault, J.L., Fiet, J., Julien, R., Dreux, C. and Canivet, J. (1980). Adrenocortical 11β-hydroxylation defect in adult women with postmenarchial onset of symptoms. *J. Clin. Endocrinol. Metab.*, **51**, 287–91

46. Birnbaum, M.D. and Rose, L.I. (1984). Late onset adrenocortical hydroxylase deficiencies associated with menstrual dysfunction. *Obstet. Gynecol.*, **63**, 445–51

47. Hurwitz, A., Brautbar, C., Milwidsky, A., Vecsei, P., Milewicz, A., Navot, D. and Rosler, A. (1985). Combined 21- and 11β-hydroxylase deficiency in familial congenital adrenal hyperplasia. *J. Clin. Endocrinol. Metab.*, **60**, 631–8

48. Bongiovanni, A.M. (1984). Congenital adrenal hyperplasia due to 3β-hydroxysteroid dehydrogenase deficiency. In New, M.I. and Levine, L.S. (eds.) *Adrenal Diseases in Childhood* (*Pediatr. Adolesc. Endocrinol.*, Vol. 13), pp. 72–82. (Basel: S. Karger)

6

Insulin resistance in polycystic ovary syndrome

J. Holte, T. Bergh and H. Lithell

A CONNECTION BETWEEN INSULIN RESISTANCE AND ANDROGENS, INDEPENDENT OF OBESITY?

A connection between hyperandrogenism and a disturbed glucose metabolism was suggested as early as 1921[1]. More recently, several investigators have reported on extreme insulin resistance and hyperandrogenism in women with acanthosis nigricans and obesity[2-4]. In these women polycystic or hyperthecotic ovaries are usually found. Hyperinsulinemia and insulin resistance have, however, been shown to be common features in polycystic ovary syndrome (PCOS), also without acanthosis nigricans[5,6]. As obesity *per se* is associated with decreased insulin sensitivity, and many women with PCOS are obese, insulin resistance in these women cannot *a priori* be attributed to their hyperandrogenism. However, hyperinsulinemia and insulin hyper-response to an oral glucose tolerance test (OGTT), suggestive of insulin resistance, was also reported in 1982 in a small group of normal-weight women with PCOS[7]. Even though several later studies have shown indications of lower insulin sensitivity in normal-weight women with PCOS compared to controls[8-12], the results have not been completely uniform. In one study, no signs of insulin resistance were found in normal-weight PCOS women[13]. In two studies, fasting hyperinsulinemia was not found in non-obese women with PCOS[10,12], whereas the same women's responses to an OGTT or an insulin clamp were indicative of lowered insulin sensitivity. Two studies[6,10] involving both ovulatory and anovulatory hyperandrogenic women showed no insulin resistance in *ovulatory* hyperandrogenic women. In a study involving both obese and non-obese women with polycystic ovaries diagnosed by means of ultrasound scanning, according to Adams' criteria[14,15], only obese PCOS women exhibited hyperinsulinemia in an intravenous glucose tolerance test and decreased insulin sensitivity in the euglycemic hyperinsulinemic insulin clamp test (Holte, Bergh, Lithell, unpublished results). Non-obese women with polycystic ovaries did not differ from weight-matched controls in any parameter of insulin sensitivity, although testosterone, androstenedione and luteinizing hormone (LH) were significantly higher and sex hormone binding globulin (SHBG) significantly lower in the polycystic ovary group. Thus, in the absence of obesity, insulin resistance is not invariably present in hyperandrogenic women.

CORRELATIONS BETWEEN INSULIN AND ANDROGENS

Significant correlations between serum androgens and both fasting insulin levels and insulin response during an oral glucose tolerance test have been found by different investigators (Table 1). Except for one study involving 14 obese women with PCOS[9], these correlations are only found when women with PCOS and controls are analyzed together; no significant correlations existed in the separate groups. Whether this discrepancy is due to small samples or whether it indicates a more indirect relationship, instead of a cause-and-effect relation, is not known. As obesity affects not only insulin levels, but also SHBG[19] and testosterone[20], resulting in an increased androgenicity parallel to increased body mass index, a correction should be made for the confounding effect of obesity, when analyzing correlations between androgens and insulin resistance. The importance of adjusting for the independent effects of obesity in this context is stressed by one large study[10] involving 50 obese and 48 non-obese women (hyperandrogenic and controls), where summed insulin response during an OGTT correlated to androstenedione and testosterone as well as to percentage of ideal body weight in the obese women, whereas in the non-obese group these correlations were not found.

CAUSALITY BETWEEN INSULIN AND ANDROGENS

There are facts supporting a cause-and-effect relationship in both directions – hyperinsulinemia as a cause of elevated androgen levels or vice versa – and there also remains a possibility that androgens and insulin are related through a common factor. In favor of that third alternative could be the

Table 1 Correlation coefficients between fasting circulating insulin and serum androgens

Investigator	n	Androstenedione	Testosterone
Burghen[5]	14	0.65**	0.71**
Chang[7]	20	0.52*	0.59*
Pasquali[9]	14	0.64**	0.46*
Shoupe[6]	19	—	0.34*
Stuart[16]	33	0.52***	0.56***
Smith[17]	17	0.57*	0.75***
Bruno[8]	33	—	0.46**
Jialal[18]	14	0.72**	0.70**
Kustin[13]	24	—	0.48*
Dunaif[10]	50†	−0.14 ns	−0.03 ns
Dunaif[10]	48‡	0.16 ns	0.23 ns

† non-obese subjects; ‡ obese subjects in one study.
* $p < 0.05$; ** $p < 0.01$; *** $p < 0.001$; ns, not significant

evidence that PCOS[21], obesity and diabetes type II are to a large extent determined by genetic factors. In further support of this third alternative is the anatomic closeness between the hypothalamic center that is believed to regulate insulin secretion[22] and the area that regulates gonadal function[23].

Several facts are in support of androgens as a cause of insulin resistance. Administration of synthetic androgens such as oxymetholone to patients with aplastic anemia induced insulin resistance[24], but it is possible that only the *oral* administration of synthetic androgens causes insulin resistance (because of a hepatotoxic effect), since parenteral synthetic androgens have not been shown to affect glucose tolerance[25,26]. Obviously, a major diabetogenic effect of natural androgens would produce a large difference in insulin sensitivity between men and women, a difference which is not found. However, expressed per kg lean body mass, insulin-mediated glucose disposal during the euglycemic clamp is 45% lower in men compared to weight-matched women[27]. Kissebah and co-workers have found a correlation between an increased waist–hip ratio, corresponding to higher androgen levels (and reduced SHBG), and insulin resistance[28]. They argued that androgens, supposedly through increased free fatty acid load to the liver, decrease liver extraction of insulin, thus causing peripheral hyperinsulinemia and insulin resistance. However, no evidence exists of a true cause-and-effect relation with androgens as the cause.

Treatment with ovarian resection[29], spironolactone[6], or combined oral contraceptive[30], resulting in decreased androgen levels in PCOS, has in some reports been shown to increase insulin sensitivity, whereas in other studies insulin resistance has persisted after oophorectomy[31,32], cyproterone acetate therapy[9], or treatment with gonadotropin releasing hormone analog[33]. It is possible that the observation time of 3–6 months in these studies was too short for a change in insulin sensitivity to take place.

Hyperinsulinemia could theoretically affect androgen levels through a direct effect on the ovaries (or indirectly through effects on the pituitary), resulting in an increased androgen production, or interfere with action or clearance of the androgenic steroids. The possibility of the last alternative is not much studied, but an interference of high insulin levels, or concomitant increased free fatty acids, with liver function and clearance of androgens is not ruled out[28]. Furthermore, there is *in vitro* support for a decreased production of SHBG in liver cells when exposed to insulin[34], a mechanism that would increase levels of biologically active testosterone.

The possibility of an ovarian effect of insulin, resulting in increased circulating androgens, is supported by several studies. Specific insulin binding sites in the human ovary have been identified[35,36]. Insulin has been shown to enhance gonadotropin-stimulated progesterone production and LH receptor induction in porcine granulosa cells[37], and to act synergistically with LH in androstenedione production from porcine theca cells[38]. In human granulosa cell incubations, insulin was shown to enhance FSH-induced aromatase activity[39]. In stroma cell incubations from normally cycling women, insulin together with LH stimulated androstenedione accumulation, whereas insulin alone could stimulate androstenedione and testosterone accumulation from both theca and stroma cell incubations from a woman with hyperandrogenism and insulin resistance[40]. Thus, insulin has been found to modulate steroid hormone biosynthesis in both animal and human *in vitro* systems.

The prevailing hypothesis is that, even though most tissues are resistant to the effects of insulin on glucose metabolism, the ovaries are still responsive and are thus being 'overstimulated' by the raised insulin levels in the insulin-resistant woman[40]. However, though much less discussed, a hypothesis that presumes that the ovary also *is* insulin resistant, would find support in the observations showing a role for insulin in the maintenance of cellular functions in granulosa cells[37] and in augmenting aromatase activity[39].

The *in vivo* androgen response to acutely increased insulin levels has been studied by several investigators, either by means of the euglycemic insulin clamp test[41-43] or by means of an OGTT[17]. Increased androstenedione levels were found in PCOS women[17,41,43], but not in normal women[43] after short-term raised insulin concentrations. No significant increases in testosterone levels were found in PCOS women[17,41,42], normal men[17] or normally cycling women[17,41-43]. One study[17] showed increases in androstenedione and dihydrotestosterone only in hyperandrogenic women with a high insulin response during OGTT, and not in those with a low insulin response. Thus, investigations of the impact of short-term increased insulin levels on androgens have yielded somewhat conflicting results. The short time of exposure to the raised insulin levels, 3–16 h, must be considered when evaluating these results.

The effect of pharmacologically *decreased* insulin levels on androgens was recently studied. By administration of diazoxide for 10 days to five obese women with PCOS, Nestler *et al.*[44] were able to show that, parallel to a markedly decreased insulin response to an OGTT, testosterone levels, but not androstenedione, fell significantly. In all patients, serum SHBG rose slightly, resulting in significantly lowered levels of non-SHBG-bound testosterone. Although the possibility that diazoxide has effects on testosterone via other mechanisms than via insulin was not evaluated, this investigation supports the hypothesis of a direct effect of insulin on androgen metabolism in the obese, hyperandrogenic woman.

CONCLUSION

The relationship between insulin sensitivity and androgens is complex. Obesity, a powerful inducer of insulin resistance, is often present in women with polycystic ovary syndrome and a confounding factor in many studies. However, it seems clear that some non-obese patients with polycystic ovary syndrome have lowered insulin sensitivity and that increased serum androgen concentrations are often found in connection with severe insulin resistance in obese women. The evidence for a direct cause-and-effect relation between insulin levels and androgens – in either direction – is not unequivocal. The existence of a common factor predisposing to both insulin hypersecretion/insulin resistance and disturbances in androgen metabolism as well as obesity remains a possible alternative.

REFERENCES

1. Achard, C. and Thiers, J. (1921). Le virilisme pilaire et son association à l'insuffisance glycolitique (Diabete à femmes de barbe). *Bull. Acad. Natle. Med. (Paris)*, **86**, 51–5
2. Kahn, C.R., Flier, J.S., Barr, R.S., Archer, J.A., Gorden, P., Martin, M.M. and Roth, J. (1976). The syndromes of insulin resistance and acanthosis nigricans: insulin receptor disorders in man. *N. Engl. J. Med.*, **294**, 739–45
3. Harrison, L.C., Dean, B., Peluso, I., Clark, S. and Ward, G. (1985). Insulin resistance, acanthosis nigricans, and polycystic ovaries associated with a circulation inhibitor of postbinding insulin action. *J. Clin. Endocrinol. Metab.*, **60**, 1047–52
4. Dunaif, A., Hoffman, A.R., Scully, R.E., Flier, J.S., Longcope, C., Levy, L.J. and Crowley, Jr, W.F. (1985). Clinical, biochemical, and ovarian morphologic features in women with acanthosis nigricans and masculinization. *Obstet. Gynecol.*, **66**, 545–52
5. Burghen, G.A., Givens, J.R. and Kitabchi, A.E. (1980). Correlation of hyperandrogenism with hyperinsulinism in polycystic ovarian disease. *J. Clin. Endocrinol. Metab.*, **50**, 113–16
6. Shoupe, D. and Lobo, R.A. (1984). The influence of androgens on insulin resistance. *Fertil. Steril.*, **41**, 385–8
7. Chang, R.J., Nakamura, R.M., Judd, H.L. and Kaplan, S.A. (1983). Insulin resistance in nonobese patients with polycystic ovarian disease. *J. Clin. Endocrinol. Metab.*, **57**, 356–9
8. Bruno, B., Poccia, G. and Fabbrini, A. (1985). Insulin resistance and secretion in polycystic ovarian disease. *J. Endocrinol. Invest.*, **8**, 443–8
9. Pasquali, R., Casimirri, F., Venturoli, S., Paradisi, R., Mattioli, L., Capelli, M., Melchionda, N. and Labo, G. (1983). Insulin resistance in patients with polycystic ovaries: its relationship to body weight and androgen levels. *Acta Endocrinol.*, **104**, 110–16
10. Dunaif, A., Graf, M., Mandeli, J., Laumas, V. and Dobrjansky, A. (1987). Characterization of groups of hyperandrogenic women with acanthosis nigricans, impaired glucose tolerance, and/or hyperinsulinemia. *J. Clin. Endocrinol. Metab.*, **65**, 499–507
11. Dunaif, A., Mandeli, J., Fluhr, H. and Dobrjansky, A. (1988). The impact of obesity and chronic hyperinsulinemia on gonadotropin release and gonadal steroid secretion in the polycystic ovary syndrome. *J. Clin. Endocrinol. Metab.*, **66**, 131–9
12. Dunaif, A., Segal, K.R., Futterweit, W. and Dobrjansky, A. (1989). Profound peripheral insulin resistance, independent of obesity, in polycystic ovary syndrome. *Diabetes*, **38**, 1165–74
13. Kustin, J., Kazer, R.R., Hoffman, D.I., Chatterton, R.T., Haan, J.N., Green, O.C. and Rebar, R.W. (1987). Insulin resistance and abnormal ovarian responses to human chorionic gonadotropin in chronically anovulatory women. *Am. J. Obstet. Gynecol.*, **157**, 1468–73
14. Franks, S., Adams, J., Mason, H. and Polson, D. (1985). Ovulatory disorders in women with polycystic ovary syndrome. *Clin. Obstet. Gynecol.*, **12**, 605–32
15. Adams, J., Polson, D.W. and Franks, S. (1986). Prevalence of polycystic ovaries in women with anovulation and idiopathic hirsutism. *Br. Med. J.*, **293**, 355–9
16. Stuart, C.A., Prince, M.J., Peters, E.J. and Meyer, III, W.J. (1987). Hyperinsulinemia and hyperandrogenemia: *in vivo* androgen response to insulin infusion. *Obstet. Gynecol.*, **69**, 921–5
17. Smith, S., Ravnikar, V.A. and Barbieri, R.L. (1987). Androgen and insulin response to an oral glucose challenge in hyperandrogenic women. *Fertil. Steril.*, **48**, 72–6
18. Jialal, I., Naiker, P., Reddi, K., Moodley, J. and Joubert, S.M. (1987). Evidence for insulin resistance in nonobese patients with polycystic ovarian disease. *J. Clin. Endocrinol. Metab.*, **64**, 1066–9
19. Plymate, S.R., Fariss, B.L., Bassett, M.M.L. and Matej, L. (1981). Obesity and its role in polycystic ovary syndrome. *J. Clin. Endocrinol. Metab.*, **52**, 1246–8
20. Wajchenberg, B.L., Acanhando, M.S., Marcondes, J.A.M., Germak, O.A., Mathor, M.B. and Kirschner, M.A. (1988). Free testosterone levels during the menstrual cycle in obese versus normal women. *Fertil. Steril.*, **51**, 535–7
21. Hague, W.M., Adams, J., Reeders, S.T., Peto, T.E.A. and Jacobs, H.S. (1988). Familial polycystic ovaries: a genetic disease? *Clin. Endocrinol.*, **29**, 593–605
22. Bray, G.A. and York, D.A. (1979). Hypothalamic and genetic obesity in experimental animals: an autonomic and endocrine hypothesis. *Physiol. Rev.*, **59**, 719–25
23. Knobil, E. (1980). The neuroendocrine control of the menstrual cycle. *Recent Prog. Horm.*

Res., **36**, 53–60

24. Woodard, T.L., Burghen, G.A., Kitabchi, A.E. and Wilimas, J.A. (1981). Glucose intolerance and insulin resistance in aplastic anemia treated with oxymetholone. *J. Clin. Endocrinol. Metab.*, **53**, 905–8

25. Lewis, L.A. and McCullagh, E.P. (1942). Carbohydrate metabolism of animals treated with methyltestosterone and testosteronepropionate. *J. Clin. Endocrinol.*, **2**, 502–8

26. Landon, J., Wynn, W. and Samols, E. (1963). The effect of anabolic steroids on blood sugar and plasma insulin levels in man. *Metabolism*, **12**, 924–9

27. Yki-Järvinen, H. (1984). Sex and insulin sensitivity. *Metabolism*, **33**, 1011–15

28. Peiris, A.N., Mueller, R.A., Struve, M.F., Smith, G.A. and Kissebah, A.H. (1987). Relationship of androgenic activity to splanchnic insulin metabolism and peripheral glucose utilization in premenopausal women. *J. Clin. Endocrinol. Metab.*, **64**, 162–9

29. Givens, J.R., Kerber, I.J., Wiser, W.L., Anderson, R.N., Coleman, S.A. and Fish, S.A. (1974). Remission of acanthosis nigricans associated with polycystic ovarian diseases and a stromal luteoma. *J. Clin. Endocrinol. Metab.*, **38**, 347–52

30. Cole, C. and Kitabchi, A.E. (1978). Remission of insulin resistance with Orthonovum in a patient with polycystic ovarian disease and acanthosis nigricans. *Clin. Res.* (Abstr.), **26**, 412

31. Annos, T. and Taymor, M.L. (1981). Ovarian pathology associated with insulin resistance and acanthosis nigricans. *Obstet. Gynecol.*, **58**, 662–4

32. Nagamani, M., Dinh, T.V. and Kelver, M.E. (1986). Hyperinsulinemia in hyperthecosis of the ovaries. *Am. J. Obstet. Gynecol.*, **154**, 384–9

33. Geffner, M.E., Kaplan, S.A., Bersch, N., Golde, D.W., Landaw, E.M. and Chang, R.J. (1986). Persistence of insulin resistance in polycystic ovarian disease after inhibition of ovarian steroid secretion. *Fertil. Steril.*, **45**, 327–33

34. Plymate, S.R., Matej, L.A., Jones, R.E. and Friedel, K.E. (1988). Inhibition of sex hormone binding globulin production in the human hepatoma (Hep G2) cell line by insulin and prolactin. *J. Clin. Endocrinol. Metab.*, **67**, 460–4

35. Poretsky, L., Smith, D., Seibel, M., Pazianos, A., Moses, A.C. and Flier, J.S. (1984). Specific insulin binding sites in human ovary. *J. Clin. Endocrinol. Metab.*, **59**, 809–11

36. Jarrett II, J.C., Ballejo, G., Tsibris, J.C.M. and Spellacy, W.N. (1985). Insulin binding to human ovaries. *J. Clin. Endocrinol. Metab.*, **60**, 460–3

37. May, J.V. and Schomberg, D.W. (1981). Granulosa cell differentiation *in vitro*: effect of insulin on growth and functional integrity. *Biol. Reprod.*, **25**, 421–3

38. Barbieri, R.L., Makris, A. and Ryan, K.J. (1983). Effects of insulin on steroidogenesis in cultured porcine ovarian theca. *Fertil. Steril.*, **40**, 237–41

39. Garzo, V.G. and Dorrington, J.H. (1984). Aromatase activity in human granulosa cells during follicular development and the modulation by follicle-stimulating hormone and insulin. *Am. J. Obstet. Gynecol.*, **148**, 657–62

40. Barbieri, R.L., Makris, A. and Ryan, K.J. (1984). Insulin stimulates androgen accumulation in incubations of human ovarian stroma and theca. *Obstet. Gynecol.*, **64**, 73–80S

41. Stuart, C.A., Prince, N.J., Peters, E.J. and Meyer, W.J. (1987). Hyperinsulinemia and hyperandrogenemia: *in vivo* response to insulin infusion. *Obstet. Gynecol.*, **69**, 921–5

42. Nestler, J.E., Clore, J.N., Strauss III, J.F. and Blackard, W.G. (1986). The effects of hyperinsulinemia on serum testosterone, progesterone, dehydroepiandrosterone sulfate, and cortisol levels in normal women and in a woman with hyperandrogenism, insulin resistance, and acanthosis nigricans. *J. Clin. Endocrinol. Metab.*, **64**, 180–4

43. Dunaif, A. and Graf, M. (1989). Insulin administration alters gonadal steroid metabolism independent of changes in gonadotrophin secretion in insulin resistant women with the polycystic ovary syndrome. *J. Clin. Invest.*, **83**, 23–9

44. Nestler, J.E., Barlascini, C.O., Matt, D.W., Steingold, K.A., Plymate, S.R., Clore, J.N. and Blackard, W.G. (1989). Suppression of serum insulin by diazoxide reduces serum testosterone levels in obese women with polycystic ovary syndrome. *J. Clin. Endocrinol. Metab.*, **68**, 1027–33

7

Obesity, hyperandrogenism and anovulation

D. Shelley and A. Dunaif

INTRODUCTION

Polycystic ovary syndrome (PCOS) is characterized by the presence of hyperandrogenism and abnormal gonadotropin secretion, producing chronic oligo- or anovulation. Stein and Leventhal's original description of PCOS included obesity as well as hirsutism and amenorrhea[1], and Yen noted that more than 80% of patients found to have PCOS were obese prior to puberty[2]. Moreover, several studies have noted that obesity is associated with elevated androgen production and an increased incidence of amenorrhea[3-5]. In this review we will use PCOS as a model for assessing the relationship between obesity, hyperandrogenism and ovulation.

These observations have led to speculation that obesity plays a role in the pathogenesis of PCOS. However, obesity occurs in only 35–60%[6,7] of women with PCOS, and, clearly, all obese women do not have hormonal disturbances. Nonetheless, there are several mechanisms by which obesity has been postulated to play a role in the development of chronic hyperandrogenic anovulation characteristic of PCOS. First, gonadal steroid feedback changes could result from obesity because of increased extraglandular aromatization of androgen to estrogen[8], and decreased sex hormone binding globulin (SHBG) levels[9]. Second, neuroendocrine abnormalities, such as a central lesion involving the putative feeding center of the ventromedial hypothalamus and the anatomically closely related neurons in the arcuate nucleus involved in pulsatile gonadotropin releasing hormone (GnRH) secretion, might explain the association of PCOS and obesity[10]. Alternatively, insulin might alter gonadotropin secretion and ovarian steroidogenesis to produce PCOS[11,12]. A correlation between hyperinsulinemia and hyperandrogenism has been shown in PCOS[13], and obese women with PCOS are significantly more hyperinsulinemic than non-obese women with PCOS[14]. Finally, obesity might be secondary to metabolic changes such as androgen-mediated increases in body weight[15], or a decrease in energy expenditure[16,17].

GONADAL STEROID FEEDBACK CHANGES

Obesity is associated with increased extragonadal aromatization of androgens to estrogens[8], decreased SHBG and increased androgen production[3,4,9]. These changes may play a role in the development of PCOS by causing chronic inappropriate estrogen feedback on the hypothalamic–pituitary axis, leading to distorted gonadotropin release and anovulation[18,19], and by increasing androgen production which may directly inhibit follicular maturation[20].

There is evidence that argues against these hypotheses. Decreased SHBG and increased androgen production occur in obese women with and without reproductive dysfunction[9,21-23]. Zhang and colleagues[21] found similarly low levels of SHBG in both ovulatory and non-ovulatory obese women. However, only the anovulatory women had increased serum androgen levels, suggesting that obesity is not the only factor contributing to chronic anovulation. These findings suggest that the putative servo-control mechanism[22], that adjusts the production rate of steroids to maintain constant levels despite an increased metabolic clearance, is not operative in obese non-cycling women.

Two recent studies have shown that the plasma levels of androgens and estrogens are similar in both lean and obese women with PCOS[7,24]. Again, these findings indicate that hyperandrogenism and anovulation can occur independent of obesity. However, there is evidence that obesity has some impact on the clinical and endocrinological abnormalities characteristic of PCOS. Obese women with PCOS have a greater prevalence of anovulation and hirsutism that non-obese women with PCOS[24]. The increased incidence of hirsutism appears related to a greater activity of the 5α-reductase enzyme system in peripheral tissues in obese women compared to lean women with PCOS[24]. Moreover, a number of studies have shown that weight reduction can improve hormonal abnormalities and restore ovulation in obese anovulatory hyperandrogenic women[25-28]. Harlass and colleagues found a significant decrease in mean luteinizing hormone (LH) and a return of ovulation in some obese anovulatory hyperandrogenic women after weight loss[27]. Similarly, Pasquali and colleagues[25] demonstrated significant decreases in testosterone (T) and mean LH levels, and improved cyclicity without changes in androstenedione (A) or dehydroepiandrosterone sulfate (DHEAS) levels in obese anovulatory hyperandrogenic women. No hormonal differences could be identified between those women who responded to weight reduction and those who did not. Therefore, although obesity may contribute to anovulation in some women with PCOS, the mechanism of this action remains unknown. Moreover, it is not possible to predict which patients will benefit from weight loss.

DISTINCT NEUROENDOCRINE DISORDER

PCOS could result from a primary central disorder of GnRH release that leads to disrupted pulsatile gonadotropin secretion, producing anovulation and hyperandrogenism[10]. We have recently shown, however, that obese and non-obese women with PCOS have similar patterns of pulsatile gonadotropin release[7]. This strongly suggests that obese women with PCOS do not have a distinct neuroendocrine disorder.

Lesions of the ventromedial hypothalamus in animals can lead to obesity and hyperinsulinemia[29]. Hence, the association of hyperinsulinemia and obesity of PCOS might be secondary to an abnormality in the ventromedial hypothalamus. Non-obese women with PCOS are hyperinsulinemic, but to a lesser degree than their obese counterparts[14]. Obesity and insulin resistance do occur without PCOS[30], and non-obese women with PCOS usually have no history of obesity (Dunaif, unpublished observations). Thus it remains possible that the gonadotropin abnormalities of PCOS, the obesity that can be associated with PCOS, and insulin resistance could represent defects at different but anatomically related loci which overlap to result in a heterogeneous disorder.

Alternatively, it is possible that other hormonal abnormalities that occur in obese PCOS women, such as hyperinsulinemia, could produce neuroendocrine changes. Indeed, obese women with PCOS have significantly increased fasting and glucose-stimulated plasma insulin levels compared to non-obese women with PCOS and obese normal women[7]. Positive linear correlations have been found between hyperinsulinemia and hyperandrogenism, leading to speculation that increased insulin levels cause PCOS[13]. Insulin can alter steroidogenesis in human and animal ovarian tissue[11,12], and supraphysiological doses of insulin can increase androgen production in vivo[31,32], but high doses of exogenous insulin have no effect on gonadotropin release in women with PCOS[31]. Moreover, we have shown that obese and non-obese women with PCOS have similar patterns of gonadotropin release and reproductive hormone levels despite significant differences in their degree of endogenous hyperinsulinemia[7]. These results suggest that physiological hyperinsulinemia does not play a major role in sustaining the hormonal abnormalities characteristic of PCOS.

METABOLIC DEFECT

If the hormonal abnormalities observed in PCOS are independent of obesity, then why is there an increased prevalence of obesity in PCOS? Hyperandrogenism can cause alterations in body composition by directly increasing muscle mass and/or stimulating food intake[15]. We found no differences, however, in either muscle or fat mass in obese PCOS as compared to obese normal women[33]. Further, not all hyperandrogenic women are obese, as evidenced by non-obese women with PCOS.

Alternatively, obesity may be related to a primary deficit in energy expenditure, increased energy intake, or both[34,35]. Ravussin and colleagues[34], in a prospective study, found that a familial decrease in total energy expenditure predicted the development of obesity. Interestingly, these subjects had low baseline resting metabolic rates, which, after weight gain, became similar to non-obese subjects. This suggests that weight gain is a way of correcting an abnormal resting metabolic rate. Similarly, Roberts and colleagues[35] found that a decrease in total energy expenditure in infants of obese women compared to infants of non-obese women was related to rapid weight gain in the first year of life. A low energy expenditure in some infants who did not develop obesity implies the existence of additional factors contributing to eventual weight gain.

A defect in energy expenditure in obese subjects may be secondary to insulin resistance. Ravussin and collegues[36] demonstrated that a defect in postprandial thermogenesis in insulin-resistant obese subjects was related to a decrease in glucose uptake and storage. Thus, impaired glucose tolerance may be the mechanism responsible for the reduced thermic effect of a meal seen in obese subjects. This defect could be corrected by restoring normal glucose uptake using increasing doses of insulin in a euglycemic glucose clamp[37]. Obesity is associated with hyperinsulinemia and insulin resistance which is exaggerated in obese women with PCOS[14,33]. Of obese women with PCOS, 20% have impaired glucose tolerance or frank diabetes[14]. Further, PCOS and obesity produce a synergistic deleterious effect on glucose homeostasis[14,33]. It would follow then that obesity in PCOS might result from a deficit in energy expenditure. We demonstrated, however, that both normal obese women and obese women with PCOS had blunted postprandial thermogenesis[38]. Thus, women with PCOS did not have altered energy expenditure when compared to normal women of similar weight and body composition, despite significantly higher basal and post-glucose load glucose levels and decreased insulin-stimulated glucose utilization. Thus, impaired thermogenesis may reflect a defect intrinsic to the obese state independent of insulin resistance. Taken together, these studies suggest that a defect in this component of energy expenditure, i.e. postprandial thermogenesis, is a result of obesity rather than a cause. Finally, there is little evidence that hyperandrogenism, or a defect in energy expenditure, are the primary causes of obesity in PCOS.

CONCLUSIONS

In conclusion, obesity is not associated with discernible changes in gonadotropin release or gonadal steroid levels in chronic hyperandrogenic anovulation. Despite significant insulin resistance, in obese women with polycystic ovary syndrome, there is no additional defect in energy expenditure. Weight reduction can improve menstrual function in some obese hyperandrogenic amenorrheic women. Thus, obesity may contribute to the hormonal abnormalities of polycystic ovary syndrome by an unknown mechanism. A common neuroendocrine change, closely linked genetic abnormalities, or obesity unmasking an underlying predisposition to anovulation could explain the association of obesity and polycystic ovary syndrome.

REFERENCES

1. Stein, I.F. and Leventhal, M.L. (1935). Amenorrhea associated with bilateral polycystic ovaries. *Am. J. Obstet. Gynecol.*, **29**, 181

2. Yen, S.S.C. (1980). The polycystic ovary syndrome. *Clin. Endocrinol.*, **12**, 177–207
3. Kirschner, M.A., Samjolik, E. and Silber, D. (1983). A comparison of androgen production and clearance in hirsute and obese women. *J. Steroid Biochem.*, **19**, 607–14
4. Samjolik, E., Kirschner, M.A., Silber, D., Schneider, G. and Ertel, N.H. (1984). Elevated production and metabolic clearance rates of androgens in morbidly obese women. *J. Clin. Endocrinol. Metab.*, **59**, 949
5. Rogers, J. and Mitchell, G.W. (1952). The relation of obesity to menstrual disturbances. *N. Engl. J. Med.*, **247**, 53–5
6. Franks, S. (1989). Polycystic ovarian syndrome: a changing perspective. *Clin. Endocrinol.*, **31**, 87–120
7. Dunaif, A., Mandeli, J., Fluhr, H. and Dobrjansky, A. (1988). The impact of obesity and chronic hyperinsulinemia on gonadotropin release and gonadal steroid secretion in the polycystic ovary syndrome. *J. Clin. Endocrinol. Metab.*, **66**, 131–9
8. Edman, C.D. and MacDonald, P.C. (1978). Effect of obesity on conversion of plasma androstenedione to estrone in ovulatory and anovulatory young women. *Am. J. Obstet. Gynecol.*, **130**, 456
9. Plymate, S.R., Fariss, B.L., Bassett, M.L. and Matej, L. (1981). Obesity and its role in polycystic ovary syndrome. *J. Clin. Endocrinol. Metab.*, **52**, 1246–8
10. Dunaif, A. and Hoffman, A.R. (1988). Insulin resitance and hyperandrogenism: clinical syndromes and possible mechanisms. In Pancheri, P. and Zichella, L. (eds.) *Biorhythms and Stress in the Physiopathology of Reproduction*, pp. 293–317. (New York: Hemisphere Publishing Corporation)
11. Barbieri, R.L., Markris, A., Randal, R.W., Daniels, G., Kistner, R.W. and Ryan, K.J. (1986). Insulin stimulates androgen accumulation in incubations of ovarian stroma obtained from women with hyperandrogenism. *J. Clin. Endocrinol. Metab.*, **62**, 904–10
12. Poretsky, L. and Kalin, M.F. (1987). The gonadotropic function of insulin. *Endocr. Rev.*, **8**, 132–9
13. Burghen, G.A., Given, J.R. and Kitabchi, A.E. (1980). Correlation of hyperandrogenism with hyperinsulinism in polycystic ovarian disease. *J. Clin. Endocrinol. Metab.*, **50**, 113–16
14. Dunaif, A., Graf, M., Mandeli, J., Laumas, V. and Dobrjansky, A. (1987). Characterization of groups of hyperandrogenic women with acanthosis nigricans, impaired glucose tolerance, and/or hyperinsulinemia. *J. Clin. Endocrinol. Metab.*, **65**, 499–507
15. Rowland, D.L., Perrings, T.S. and Thomas, J.A. (1980). Comparison of androgenic effects on food intake and body weight in adult rats. *Physiol. Behav.*, **24**, 205–9
16. James, W.P.T. and Trayhurn, P. (1981). Thermogenesis and obesity. *Br. Med. Bull.*, **37**, 43–8
17. Jung, R.T., Setty, P.S. and James, W.T.T. (1979). Reduced thermogenesis in obesity. *Nature (London)*, **279**, 322–3
18. Yen, S.S.C., Chaney, C. and Judd, H.L. (1976). Functional aberration in the polycystic ovary syndrome: a consideration of the pathogenesis. In James, V.H.T., Serio, M. and Gusti, G. (eds.) *The Endocrine Function of the Human Ovary*, p.373. (New York: Academic Press)
19. Rebar, R., Judd, H.L., Yen, S.S.C., Rakoff, J., Vandenberg, G. and Naftolin, F. (1976). Characterization of the inappropriate gonadotropin secretion in polycystic ovary syndrome. *J. Clin. Invest.*, **57**, 1320–9
20. Louvet, J.P., Harman, S.M., Schreiber, J.R. and Ross, G.T. (1975). Evidence for a role of androgens in follicular maturation. *Endocrinology*, **97**, 366–72
21. Zhang, Y., Ster, B. and Rebar, R.W. (1984). Endocrine comparison of obese menstruating and amenorrheic women. *J. Clin. Endocrinol. Metab.*, **58**, 1077–83
22. Kurtz, B.R., Givens, J.R., Kamindr, S., Stevens, M.D., Karas, J.G., Bittle, J.B., Judge, D. and Kitabchi, A. (1987). Maintenance of normal circulating levels of Δ^4 androstenedione and dehydroepiandrosterone in simple obesity despite increased metabolic clearance rates: evidence for a servo-control mechanism. *J. Clin. Endocrinol. Metab.*, **64**, 1261–7
23. Hossenian, A.H., Kim, M.H. and Rosenfield, R.L. (1976). Obesity and oligomenorrhea are associated with hyperandrogenism independent of hirsutism. *J. Clin. Endocrinol. Metab.*, **42**, 765–9
24. Kiddy, D.S., Sharp, P.S., White, D.M., Scanlon, M.F., Mason, H.D., Bray, C.S., Polson, D.W., Reed, M.J. and Franks, S. (1989). Differences in clinical and endocrine features between obese and nonobese subjects with polycystic ovary syndrome: an analysis of 263 consecutive cases. *Clin. Endocrinol.*, in press

25. Pasquali, R., Antemucci, D., Casimirri, F., Venturoli, S., Paradisi, R., Fabbri, R., Balestra, V., Melchionda, N. and Barbara, L. (1989). Clinical and hormonal characteristics of obese amenorrheic hyperandrogenic women before and after weight loss. *J. Clin. Endocrinol. Metab.*, **68**, 173–9

26. Bates, G.W. and Whitworth, N.S. (1982). Effect of body weight reduction on plasma androgens in obese, infertile women. *Fertil. Steril.*, **38**, 406–9

27. Harlass, F.E., Plymate, S.R., Fariss, B.L. and Belts, R.P. (1984). Weight loss is associated with correction of gonadotropin and sex steroid abnormalities in the obese anovulatory female. *Fertil. Steril.*, **42**, 469–52

28. Mitchell, G.W. and Rogers, J. (1953). The influence of weight reduction on amenorrhea in obese women. *N. Engl. J. Med.*, **249**, 835–7

29. Bray, G.A. and York, D.A. (1979). Hypothalamic and genetic obesity in experimental animals: an autonomic and endocrine hypothesis. *Physiol. Rev.*, **59**, 719–809

30. Bar, R.S., Gorden, P., Roth, J., Kahn, C.R. and Demeyts, P. (1976). Fluctuations in the affinity and concentrations of insulin receptors on circulating monocytes of obese patients: effects of starvation, refeeding, and dieting. *J. Clin. Endocrinol. Metab.*, **58**, 1123–35

31. Dunaif, A. and Graf, M. (1989). Insulin administration alters gonadal steroid metabolism independent of changes in gonadotropin secretion in insulin-resistant women with polycystic ovary syndrome. *J. Clin. Invest.*, **83**, 23–9

32. Stuart, G.A., Prince, M.J., Peters, E.J. and Meyer, W.J. (1987). Hyperinsulinemia and hyperandrogenemia: *in vitro* androgen response to insulin infusion. *Obstet. Gynecol.*, **69**, 921–5

33. Dunaif, A., Segal, K.R., Futterweit, W. and Dobrjansky, A. (1989). Profound peripheral insulin resistance, independent of obesity, in polycystic ovary syndrome. *Diabetes*, **38**, 1165–74

34. Ravussin, E., Lillioja, S., Knowler, W.C., Christin, L., Freymond, D., Abbot, W.G.H., Boyce, V., Howard, B.V. and Bogardus, C. (1988). Reduced rate of energy expenditure as a risk factor for body-weight gain. *N. Engl. J. Med.*, **318**, 467–72

35. Roberts, S.B., Savage, J., Coward, W.A., Chew, B. and Lucas, A. (1988). Energy expenditure and intake in infants born to lean and overweight mothers. *N. Engl. J. Med.*, **318**, 461–6

36. Ravussin, E., Bogardus, C., Schwartz, R.S., Robbins, D.C., Wolfe, R.R., Horton, E.S., Danforth, E. and Sims, E.A.H. (1983). Thermic effect of infused glucose and insulin in man. *J. Clin. Invest.*, **72**, 893–902

37. Ravussin, E., Acheson, K.J., Vernet, O., Danforth, E. and Jequir, E. (1985). Evidence that insulin resistance is responsible for the decreased thermic effect of glucose in human obesity. *J. Clin. Invest.*, **76**, 1268–73

38. Segal, K.R. and Dunaif, A. (1989). Resting metabolic rate and postprandial thermogenesis in polycystic ovarian syndrome. *Int. J. Obesity*, **14**, 559–67

SECTION 2

Induction of ovulation

8

Treatment of an underlying disease in chronic hyperandrogenic anovulation

M.H. Birkhäuser

What is the origin of chronic hyperandrogenic anovulation (CHA)? This question has been debated intensely since the first description of the polycystic ovary syndrome (PCOS) by Stein and Leventhal more than 50 years ago[1]. Traditionally, within CHA, we are used to distinguishing two main groups. Following Yen[2], we may speak of the classical form of CHA without an underlying disease (PCOS) and of the CHA with an underlying disease, also called PCO-like syndrome (Table 1).

The classical form comprises again three pathophysiological subgroups:

(1)   CHA by ovarian origin,

(2)   CHA by central (hypothalamic) origin,

(3)   CHA induced by an abnormal adrenarche.

There are strong arguments suggesting that an intraovarian defect might be the most important cause of classical PCOS. But the hypothesis of a

Table 1   Classification of chronic hyperandrogenic anovulation

---

'Classical' chronic hyperandrogenic anovulation
Ovarian origin
Central (hypothalamic) origin
Abnormal adrenarche

Chronic hyperandrogenic anovulation secondary to an underlying disease
Congenital adrenal hyperplasia (CAH)
   classical form
   non-classical (late-onset, adult-onset) form
Cushing's syndrome
Ovarian hyperthecosis; hilar cell hyperplasia
Androgen producing tumors
   ovarian
   adrenal
Thyroid dysfunction (hyper-/hypothyroidism)
Obesity
Hyperprolactinemia

hypothalamic origin as well as the theory of an initial abnormal adrenarche are supported by careful studies such as the reports of the group of Yen[2] and the observations of Zumoff and colleagues[3]. However, these three main causes of classical CHA lead to the same clinical picture and to the same pathophysiological vicious circle, so that it is mostly impossible to decide where the syndrome started from. In addition, at the stage of the full-blown clinical picture, our therapeutic possibilities are the same for all subgroups of classical CHA.

This is different for patients suffering from CHA secondary to an underlying disease. Although the clinical picture might be identical, these women have to be treated in a specific way, and most of the patients can be treated successfully. It is therefore of utmost importance to recognize an underlying disease in CHA. The following conditions may lead to the clinical picture of CHA: congenital adrenal hyperplasia (classical form/late-onset or non-classical form); Cushing's syndrome; ovarian hyperthecosis, androgen-producing tumors; thyroid dysfunction; obesity; hyperprolactinemia.

The aim of the present review is to summarize the therapeutic approach in these underlying diseases leading to CHA. For better understanding, some clinical data and diagnostic procedures have to be recalled. Treatment of obesity by weight reduction and the administration of prolactin inhibitors in CHA will be omitted because this volume includes separate reviews on these two aspects. Therefore, the underlying endocrine adrenal, ovarian and thyroid causes will be the main topic of this chapter. By its incidence, congenital adrenal hyperplasia or adrenogenital syndrome is the most important representative of this group.

CONGENITAL ADRENAL HYPERPLASIA

Congenital adrenal hyperplasia (CAH) is one of the most frequent heredo-pathies. As long as 40 years ago, it had been suspected that in some patients a variant of classical congenital adrenal hyperplasia might be the underlying disease for CHA[4]. Mostly, CAH is due to a deficiency in 21-hydroxylase (90% of patients). The incidence of classical 21-hydroxylase-deficiency is variable and lies between 1 : 5000 and 1 : 15 000[5]. In Caucasians, the incidence of heterozygous carriers of the classical type is about 1 : 100[6]. This adrenal anomaly is linked to the HLA complex situated on the short arm of chromosome 6 and is inherited as a monogenic autosomal recessive trait[6-8]. Strikingly more frequent than the classical CAH is the late-onset or adult-onset or non-classical CAH[4]. Today, it is accepted that there exist several allelic variants at the 21-hydroxylase locus[9,10]. Three alleles for 21-hydroxylase deficiency are postulated: 'normal', 'mild' and 'severe'. Patients from the non-classical (late-onset, attenuated, acquired) form of CHA are homozygous for the mild allele or carrier of one mild and one severe allele[9,11,12]. Cryptic adrenal hyperplasia is asymptomatic, but is biochemically indistinguishable from the symptomatic late-onset form[13,14]. About 10% of the patients have the much rarer deficiencies in 11β-hydroxylase or in 3β-hydroxysteroid dehydrogenase. 11β-hydroxylase deficiency exists in the classical and in a non-classical, milder form. Following some authors, the incidence of 3β-dehydrogenase deficiency may reach 12.9% in hirsute women[15-19]. Because, unlike 21- and 11β-hydroxylase deficiency, this genetically transmitted enzymatic deficiency concerns both the adrenal and the ovary, baseline plasma 17-hydroxypregnenolone, dehydroepiandrosterone and dehydroepiandrosterone sulfate levels are elevated in the moderate form, as may be plasma testosterone and androstenedione. In milder forms, the elevation of the baseline values might not be very characteristic, so that, as in 21-hydroxylase deficiency, a stimulation test by adrenocorticotropic hormone (ACTH) has to be used. The diagnosis of 21-hydroxylase deficiency can be obtained prenatally[11]. Prenatal diagnosis is more difficult for 11β-hydroxylase deficiency.

In this volume, more information about the epidemiology and the diagnostic approach of CAH is given by Dr Mary New (Chapter 5).

Classical congenital adrenal hyperplasia

The treatment of classical congenital adrenal hyperplasia consists of the substitution of the missing glucocorticoids whose synthesis is reduced by the enzymatic deficiency.

In childhood, the preference is given to hydrocortisone. The dosage lies between 15 and 25 mg/m^2 per day and should be adapted individually. This amount of hydrocortisone has to be divided into three doses per day. Salt losers should receive in addition 0.05–0.1 mg fludrocortisone per day.

In adult patients, hydrocortisone may be replaced by prednisone, 5–7.5 mg/day, or by dexamethasone, 0.5–0.75 mg/day. However, there are some patients needing higher dosages to reach regular ovulatory cycles.

The monitoring of the substitution comprises, on the one hand, the clinical aspect of the patient. The appearance of Cushingoid symptoms points to an overdosage of glucocorticoids. On the other hand, the decrease of the elevated cortisol precursors typical for each type of the different enzymatic deficiencies and the normalization of the androgen secretion are good parameters for the adjustment of the treatment. Morning serum cortisol should be monitored to detect and avoid oversuppression. The latter is unlikely, if morning serum cortisol is maintained at or above 2 μg/dl[20].

In a pregnancy where a classical form of CAH might be suspected by the genotype of the parents, treatment with dexamethasone should be recommended during the first trimester to prevent virilization of the fetus[21].

Late-onset congenital adrenal hyperplasia

Late-onset or non-classical congenital adrenal hyperplasia cannot be distinguished clinically from classical chronic hyperandrogenic anovulation or from idiopathic hirsutism. Table 2[22] presents an overview of the incidence of late-onset CAH due to a deficiency in 21-hydroxylase in different

Table 2 Incidence of non-classical congenital adrenal hyper-plasia[22]

	Non-classical disease	Heterozygous carrier
Eastern European Jews	1 in 30	1 in 3
Hispanics	1 in 40	1 in 4
Yugoslavs	1 in 50	1 in 5
Italians	1 in 333	1 in 9
Others	1 in 1000	1 in 14

populations. The highest incidence is found in Eastern European Jews followed by Hispanics, Yugoslavs and Italians. In a population not related to one of these four groups, the incidence is one patient in 1000 people, the incidence of the carriers being one carrier in 14 people. Depending on the origin and the family history of the patient, late-onset or non-classical CAH might therefore be a frequent underlying disease in CHA.

Although, as mentioned above, the clinical presentation is highly variable, non-classical CAH induces characteristic cosmetic problems such as acne or hirsutism. The incidence of non-classical 21-hydroxylase deficiency in hirsute women is estimated to be between 1.2 and 20%[23-28]. The mean incidence calculated from these studies is 5%[12]. A reliable diagnostic method based on the measurement of 17α-hydroxyprogesterone following ACTH-stimulation has been described by New et al.[29]. The different methods using stimulated hormone values have recently been critically discussed by Brodie and Wentz[12].

Late-onset CAH is responsible for a significantly lower pregnancy rate in women desiring to have children and, if pregnancy occurs, by a high abortion rate[30]. In the literature, abortion rates up to 90% are mentioned in patients suffering from late-onset CAH[31].

As in the classical form, the treatment consists in late-onset CAH in the administration of glucocorticoids. Glucocorticoids aim at a return of regular ovulatory cycles and a decrease of the clinical signs of androgenization by a reduction of cortisol precursors following the suppression of endogenous ACTH[23,24,26,32-35]. Recommended are prednisone, 5–7.5 mg/day, or dexamethasone, 0.25–0.75 mg/day. If necessary, the dosage might be increased to 10 mg of prednisone or 1 mg of dexamethasone. To avoid oversuppression and Cushingoid side-effects, the lowest effective dosage should be used. The glucocorticoid should always be administered at night because of the well-known circadian rhythm of ACTH exhibiting the highest values in the early morning hours.

In general, glucocorticoids have been used in chronic hyperandrogenic anovulation since 1953[4]. The reported ovulation rate varies in the literature between 45 and 66%, the pregnancy rate between 17 and 44%[36-42]. The best results are reached in patients with an excess of adrenal androgens, as is the case in CAH[31]. The lowest success rate is observed, as expected, in patients with pure ovarian androgen excess although glucocorticoids may be able to suppress androgens of ovarian as well as of adrenal origin[39,43-46]. Glucocorticoids do not exert any teratogenic effect[36,47]. If both parents are heterozygotes for the 21-hydroxylase-'severe'-allele, the risk of having a child presenting the classical form of CAH is 25%, a risk that indicates a prophylactic dexamethasone treatment.

Because of the unusually high abortion rate in CAH[30,31], Sarris and colleagues treated a series of patients suffering from late-onset CAH by glucocorticoids (prednisone 2.5–10 mg/day) and reduced the incidence of spontaneous abortions from 91% to 9.4%[31]. Steinberger and colleagues[48] compared the abortion rate in patients with chronic hyperandrogenic anovulation following the administration of prednisone to the following ovulation induction by clomiphene. Whereas the abortion rate was still elevated with clomiphene, there was no significant difference between prednisone-treated patients and healthy controls. The same authors compared the incidence of twins in prednisone- and in clomiphene-treated women. Again, the incidence is clearly higher in clomiphene-treated patients (5.9%) than in prednisone-treated women (1.3%). This difference is statistically significant. These two parameters, abortion rate and incidence of twins, demonstrate that the suppression of an excessive androgen production by glucocorticoids is a strikingly more physiological approach than the induction of follicular maturation by clomiphene in patients with elevated adrenal androgen secretion. Therefore, anovulatory patients suffering from non-classical CAH should be treated preferentially by prednisone or dexamethasone and not by clomiphene. The normalization of the adrenal androgen secretion by glucocorticoids ameliorates the intraovarian androgen milieu and enables the ovary to start again with spontaneous follicular maturation. In CAH, the addition of clomiphene is reserved for patients in whom glucocorticoids alone have failed to restore normal follicular maturation[41].

In patients not desiring pregnancy, the administration of a hormonal contraceptive pill can be helpful. The new low-dosed pills containing a progestogen of the third generation (desogestrel, gestodene, norgestimate) act essentially through the elevation of sex hormone binding globulin (SHBG) to lower the free fraction of SHBG-bound androgens. In addition, there is a suppression of the ovarian steroid secretion. However, the clinical improvement in hirsutism induced by a normal birth control pill is mostly poor. Therefore, the choice of an antiandrogen, such as cyproterone acetate or chlormadinone acetate instead of a classical progestogen, should be recommended because of its direct effect on the peripheral androgen receptor[49,50]. As an alternative, spironolactone can be used in hirsutism because of its well-known antiandrogenic action.

CUSHING'S SYNDROME

The incidence of Cushing's syndrome is about ten patients per one million people. We distinguish between the central form, called also Cushing's disease, the peripheral form and the form secondary to an ectopic production of ACTH.

Cushing's disease represents about 60% of all Cushing patients. It is due to a hypothalamic excess production of corticotropin releasing factor (CRF) or to an excess of ACTH production by an adenoma of the pituitary. This disease is about 9 times more common in women than in males[51-54].

The peripheral form, due to an adrenal adenoma or carcinoma, comprises about 25% of the patients. Its incidence is the same in females and in males[51-54].

In about 15%, the origin of the disease is the tumoral ectopic production of ACTH, in half of the cases by a bronchus carcinoma. This form is 10 times more frequent in the male.

Clinical picture[51-57] (Table 3)

The onset of Cushing's syndrome may be slow and gradual or rapid. The first symptom in women is usually the appearance of oligomenorrhea and anovulation progressing to amenorrhea. This explains the fact that patients with Cushing's syndrome are not infrequently addressed to a center of gynecological endocrinology for investigation of menstrual irregularities combined with hirsutism.

Obesity is usual, although typically arms and legs remain thin. However, in about 50%, the obesity is generally distributed. Early signs are lassitude, loss of muscular strength and emotional disturbances. Backache and bone pain, due to osteoporosis, are frequent. Thromboembolic phenomena are common. There is an increase of Factors VIII, V and prothrombin. There might be an immunosuppression leading to opportunistic infections. At the physical examination, the patient exhibits characteristically a round face

Table 3 Cushing's syndrome: clinical picture[55-57]

	Incidence (%)		
	Ref. 55	*Ref. 56*	*Ref. 57*
Physical changes			
Round facies/full cheeks ('moon face')	88	88	88
(Central) obesity	86	97	90
Facial plethora	77		
Hirsutism	73	73	79
Broad purple striae	60	56	68
Hemorrhagic diathesis	59	62	63
Osteoporosis	58	50	64
Buffalo hump	54	54	
Acne	54	21	
Ecchymosis	52	62	63
Functional disturbances			
Hypertension	85	94	80
Amenorrhea	77	77	80
Muscular weakness	67	29	
Ankle edemas	57	50	56
Mental changes	46	62	
Difficulty in wound healing	35		
Backache/bone pains	54	43	50

with full cheeks ('moon-face'), facial plethora, a buffalo hump, a thin, atrophic skin, broad purple striae (particularly at the lower abdomen and the hips) and easy bruising. In women, hirsutism, acne and alopecia are common; acanthosis nigricans may be seen. However, true virilization is rare. In adrenal tumors producing cortisol and androgens, the excess androgen secretion may blunt the catabolic protein loss seen in pure Cushing's syndrome, so that the muscular mass is preserved and the typical striae are missing. In this condition, pronounced hirsutism and virilization may appear. Cushingoid habitus and masculinization are usually missing in hyperadrenocorticism secondary to an ectopic ACTH production.

Diagnostic approach (Table 4)

To choose the correct treatment in Cushing's syndrome, the origin of the excessive steroid secretion has first to be determined.

The classical screening tests used in the case of suspicion of Cushing's syndrome are the measurement of the 24-hour urinary excretion of free cortisol, the short dexamethasone suppression test (overnight 1 mg dexa-methasone suppression test) and the late-afternoon serum level of cortisol. Whereas in the normal non-obese subject, ACTH and cortisol are suppressed by the administration of 1 mg of dexamethasone at midnight, that is rarely the case in the presence of Cushing's syndrome. In patients with a borderline result, the 2-day low-dose dexamethasone test is performed. The low-dose long dexamethasone test using 4×0.5 mg dexamethasone/day for 2 days has the advantage that there are clearly less false-positive answers than in the classical short or overnight test. A normal response excludes Cushing's syndrome. False-positive responses may be due to an acute or chronic illness, to a hyperestrogenic state (pregnancy, pill), to obesity, depression, alcoholism or phenytoin therapy.

The high-dose dexamethasone test (4×2 mg/day for 2 days) usually suppresses the central, but not the peripheral form due to an adrenal tumor, and rarely the Cushing's syndrome due to an ectopic ACTH production. Faster, simpler and therefore more reliable is the high-dose overnight dexamethasone suppression test using a single dexamethasone dose of 8 mg orally, administered at 11 p.m. Plasma cortisol is measured at 8 a.m. the following morning. In Cushing's disease, serum cortisol levels are reduced to less than 50% in 95% of patients. This high-dose overnight test allows, therefore, a rapid differential diagnosis between Cushing's disease and patients with cortisol-producing adrenal adenomas or carcinomas or with ectopic ACTH production. However, the results may be false-negative.

A further way to distinguish between adrenal adenoma, the central form (Cushing's disease) and ectopic ACTH production is the determination of serum ACTH levels. ACTH levels are suppressed and therefore low in the presence of an adrenal adenoma or carcinoma. ACTH may be normal or slightly elevated in the central form, whereas ACTH levels are mostly greater than 100 pg/ml in ectopic ACTH production by a neoplasm. However, there is considerable overlapping between basal ACTH levels in the central form

Table 4 Diagnostic procedures in Cushing's syndrome

Screening tests

(1) 24-hour-urinary excretion of free cortisol:
normal: 20–40 μg = 55–250 nmol/24 h

(2) Late-afternoon serum cortisol level:
normal: serum cortisol < 15 μg/100 ml (< 400 nmol/1)

(3) Overnight 1 mg dexamethasone suppression test
normal: serum cortisol (day 2) < 5 μg/100 ml (< 140 nmol/1)

Differential diagnosis of hypercortisolism
Two-day low-dose dexamethasone test
Method:
0.5 mg dexamethasone orally every 6 h for 2 days
measurement of morning serum cortisol and 24 h urinary excretion of free cortisol

Response in patients without Cushing's syndrome on day two:
morning serum cortisol < 5 μg/dl (140 nmol/1)
24 h excretion of free cortisol: < 25 μg/day (70 nmol/day)

About 95% of patients with Cushing's syndrome have an abnormal response. False-positive results are rare (see text).

Overnight high-dose dexamethasone test
Method:
blood sampling for baseline morning serum cortisol
8 mg dexamethasone orally at 11 p.m.
measurement of serum cortisol at 8 a.m. on the following morning

Reduction of serum cortisol on day two:
to less than 50%: suspicion of Cushing's disease*
little or no reduction: suspicion of adrenal tumors or ectopic ACTH syndrome

*95% of patients with Cushing's disease will suppress to < 50%.

Two-day high-dose dexamethasone test
Method:
2 mg dexamathasone orally every 6 h for 2 days
measurement of morning serum cortisol and 24 h urinary excretion of free cortisol before and on the second day of dexamethasone administration

Reduction of urine free cortisol and serum cortisol on day two:
to less than 50%: suspicion of Cushing's disease*
little or no reduction: suspicion of adrenal tumors or ectopic ACTH production

*15–30% of patients with Cushing's disease are false-negative.

Further steps (*see text*)
Cushing's disease/ectopic ACTH-production: determination of serum ACTH; CRF-test, imaging by CT or magnetic resonance; selective venous sampling;

Adrenal tumor: CT; ultrasonography, iodocholesterol scanning

(Cushing's disease) and in ectopic ACTH production, particularly in the range between 100 and 250 pg ACTH per ml[58].

Following Chrousos *et al.*[59], the CRF test can help to differentiate the origin of ACTH production. Whereas in the central form, CRF provokes an excessive ACTH response, CRF is not able to induce a further increase of the already high ACTH level in ectopic ACTH production.

After the definite biochemical diagnosis, the tumor has to be localized. To localize the pituitary ACTH-producing adenoma, there are two different ways: imaging by computer-assisted tomography (CT) scan or magnetic resonance (MRI), and selective venous catheterization. In small microadenomas of the pituitary, neuroradiological studies by CT scan or MRI are often not successful. In these patients (40%) with an unclear or even normal neuroradiological result, selective venous sampling has to be done. Samples for determination of ACTH are collected from the inferior petrosal sinuses, from the venae iugulares and (in case of suspicion of ectopic ACTH production) from other sites and compared with simultaneous peripheral vein samples. To localize an adrenal tumor, CT scan, ultrasonography and isotope scanning with iodocholesterol are used. In the rare small adrenal tumors of less than 2 cm diameter, arteriography and phlebography are required.

Treatment

Untreated Cushing's syndrome may be fatal secondary to sustained hypercortisolism and its complications such as hypertension, cardiovascular or thromboembolic disease, stroke, diabetes mellitus and increased susceptibility to infections. Without treatment, about 50% of the patients will die within 5 years. However, in the presence of an adrenal cancer or ectopic ACTH production, death is more likely to be the direct consequence of the underlying tumor.

Modern treatment of Cushing's syndrome consists in the normalization of cortisol secretion by removal or correction of the primary lesion without destruction of the surrounding normal pituitary or adrenal tissue. An optimal treatment depends on a precise definition of the origin of hypercortisolism.

Surgical treatment

Cushing's disease In the central form (Cushing's disease), the treatment of choice is the selective transsphenoidal adenomectomy. In smaller adenomas, this micro-neurosurgical approach allows the extirpation of the adenoma without destruction of the surrounding pituitary and therefore without successive panhypopituitarism. In microadenomas, normalization of cortisol secretion without alteration of pituitary function is reported in 80–90%[60]. Without going into details, the necessity of a transient postoperative glucocorticoid substitution has to be underlined. The transfrontal approach is reserved for macroadenomas, particularly for tumors with extrasellar growth. In this group, a normal endocrine function can be obtained in about 50%[60].

In some patients, postoperative radiotherapy might be necessary. In inoperable situations, medical treatment is able to ameliorate the clinical condition. Because of the risk of development of Nelson's syndrome (30–40%), bilateral adrenalectomy should be used only as a last resort[61]. Nelson's syndrome, probably the consequence of central disinhibition, is characterized by a pituitary tumor, an increase of pigmentation of the skin and of the mucosa and high plasma levels of ACTH and melanocyte stimulating hormone (MSH). It cannot be prevented by preoperative irradiation of the pituitary, but irradiation is used to reduce the growth of the tumor. The treatment of established Nelson's syndrome is neurosurgical, the approach mostly transfrontal because the tumor may have extended above the diaphragma sellae. Implantation of radioactive isotopes may allow the control of the disease[62].

Peripheral form (adrenal tumor)   In the presence of an adrenal tumor, the treatment of choice is the unilateral adrenalectomy. Again, the necessity of a transient postoperative glucocorticoid substitution has to be underlined. In inoperable adrenal carcinomas, hypercortisolism can be positively influenced and sometimes stabilized by medical treatment.

Ectopic ACTH production   In ectopic ACTH production, the choice of treatment is determined by the nature and the staging of the underlying tumor, frequently a bronchus carcinoma. It is the nature of the primary tumor too that decides upon the prognosis which is usually reserved in the presence of an ectopic ACTH production. Inoperable cases might be considerably ameliorated by medical treatment.

Medical treatment

If no complete extirpation of the endocrine-active tissue is possible, for instance in adrenal carcinoma, or if the patient has to be prepared for the operation by lowering his cortisol levels, medical treatment can be adopted.

The substances used have mostly a specific affinity to steroid-producing cells and inhibit the growth of tumoral cells. The classical drugs are 2,4'-dichlorodiphenyldichloroethane (mitotane), aminogluthetimide and metyrapone. However, the side-effects of these drugs may be considerable. As an alternative, ketoconazole may be used.

Mitotane is the most powerful of the four and is able to destroy the adrenal cortex. It has a specific inhibitory action on the activity of the adrenal cortex. The classical indication is the antineoplastic use in inoperable adrenocortical tumors. The recommended starting dose is 4×0.5 g/day orally, augmented progressively to 8–12 g/day up to tolerance. The maximum tolerated dose may vary from 1 to 16 g/day. In Cushing's disease, mitotane has been used as an alternative to transsphenoidal adenomectomy and has been combined with hypophyseal irradiation[63,64]. Remission can be induced in about 80% of the patients receiving mitotane alone[63] and in up to 100% of the patients treated by mitotane in combination with irradiation[63-65], but relapse occurs in 50–60%. Remission can be maintained by very low doses such as 500 mg twice weekly[64]. Unfortunately, side-effects are frequent (nausea, vomiting, anorexia, sometimes diarrhea). In about 40%, central toxicity and neuromuscular disturbances with dizziness, vertigo, sedation, lethargy, and mental depression are observed. Permanent brain damage has been reported with prolonged use. Other side-effects are ocular problems and allergic reactions.

Therefore, this conservative therapeutic approach should not be used in operable Cushing's disease except on special indication[65,66]. The opinion prevails that the treatment of choice of Cushing's disease is neurosurgery. In contrast, 'medical adrenalectomy' with mitotane might be an excellent approach in inoperable pituitary[65,67] or adrenal tumors or ectopic ATCH syndrome. Combination with aminogluthetimide or metyrapone may allow a decrease of the dosage used and therefore a diminution of the side-effects. Replacement therapy with corticosteroids is usually required during mitotane administration. If the treatment is continued for more than 6 months, about 50% of the patients need permanent substitution therapy thereafter because of definite 'medical adrenalectomy'[63]. However, aldosterone production may continue unaltered[68].

Aminogluthetimide inhibits the adrenal corticosteroid secretion by preventing the conversion of cholesterol to pregnenolone. In addition, by its action on the peripheral aromatase, it blocks the conversion of androgens to estrogens. Side-effects include drowsiness, ataxia, lethargy, gastrointestinal and hepatic disturbances, fever, skin rashes and bone marrow depression. Other rare adverse reactions have been reported. In Cushing's syndrome, the recommended starting dose is 250 mg twice daily orally, increased to approximately 2 g/day. Simultaneously, 20 mg of cortisol or 25 mg of cortisone should be administered prophylactically to avoid symptomatic hypocortisolism. If dexamethasone is used, large doses (3 mg or more daily) have to be employed because aminogluthetimide accelerates the metabolism of dexamethasone. The extent of the adrenal blockade can be controlled by the measurement of plasma dehydroepiandrosterone (DHEA).

The blockade is complete if the values of DHEA fall below the limit of detection. As soon as this stage has been reached, the dose of aminogluthetimide can be reduced. The minimum effective dose may be as low as 1 g/day[69], an amount that is usually not toxic. The indication should be limited to inoperable adrenal carcinoma and to ectopic ACTH syndrome. However, aminogluthetimide may be used in patients with Cushing's disease awaiting the results of radiotherapy[68,70].

Metyrapone is not an effective therapeutic when given by itself because it produces only partial inhibition of steroid synthesis and because it induces overproduction of deoxycorticosterone, known to provoke hypertension. Metryapone has been recommended for combined use together with aminogluthetimide to ensure complete pharmacological blockade[70]. By using smaller doses of each substance than would be needed if they were given individually, the incidence of side-effects is reduced. By the administration of 4×250 mg metyrapone per day orally, the daily amount of aminogluthetimide needed for control of Cushing's syndrome can be reduced to 500–750 mg. Corticosteroid (cortisol, cortisone, dexamethasone) and sometimes mineralocorticoid (fludrocortisone) substitution has to be administered prophylactically[69,70].

Ketoconazole is an imidazole antifungal agent inhibiting the ergosterol synthesis of the cell membranes. Since, in addition, high doses of ketoconazole (200–400 mg four times daily) inhibit the synthesis of adrenal and testicular steroids, it has been investigated in the treatment of different endocrinopathies such as Cushing's syndrome, hirsutism and precocious puberty. It has been used with good results in Cushing's disease[71], in adrenal carcinoma[72] and in ectopic ACTH syndrome[73]. Adverse effects include gastrointestinal disturbances, rash, pruritus, headache, dizziness, somnolence and thrombocytopenia. Gynecomastia and hepatitis are rare.

THYROID DYSFUNCTION

Thyroid dysfunction may also lead to chronic hyperandrogenic anovulation. The pathophysiological connections between thyroid function and the gonadal axis are situated on two levels[2]:

(1) On the hypothalamo-hypophyseal level a common regulatory mechanism for thyroid stimulating hormone (TSH) and for prolactin exists. Primary hypothyroidism induces a rise in thyrotropin releasing hormone (TRH) that stimulates not only TSH, but also prolactin.

(2) On the hepatic level, the thyroid hormones influence the formation of sex hormone binding globulin. Hyperthyroidism leads to an increase, hypothyroidism to a decrease of binding proteins.

Hyperthyroidism

There are two ways known in hyperthyroidism to favor the incidence of chronic hyperandrogenic anovulation. The increase of SHBG provokes a decrease of the metabolic clearance rate of estrogens and androgens[74,75]. Therefore, plasma testosterone concentration is elevated. The consequence is an increased conversion of testosterone to androstenedione and an increased peripheral production of estrogens[76,77]. Furthermore, the 2-hydroxylase activity increases in hyperthyroidism, leading to a rise of the production of catecholestrogens[78]. Both mechanisms induce a chronic elevation of estrogens and may result in an inappropriate feedback and in an increased, inadequate LH production, explaining the CHA in hyperthyroidism[76].

Treatment

In *toxic adenoma*, the treatment of choice in younger patients is the surgical enucleation of the hot nodule. In older patients, the administration of radioiodine is preferred. Antithyroid drugs may be used prior to surgery or after administration of radioiodine until its full effect is reached.

In *Grave's disease*, the initial treatment is mostly the administration of antithyroid drugs such as carbimazole or propyl-thio-uracil. In a second stage, radioiodine or surgery might be chosen, depending on the size of the tumor, the age of the patient and the importance of the hyperfunction.

Treatment of hyperthyroidism has to be monitored by TSH, determined by an ultrasensitive assay, or by the response of TSH to TRH. Typical for untreated hyperthyroidism is the absence of any TSH response to TRH. Any treatment of hyperthyroidism should aim at the normalization of the TRH test. Today, an ultrasensitive TSH assay may be used for intermediate treatment controls.

Hypothyroidism

In hypothyroidism, the decrease of SHBG induces an increase of the metabolic clearance rate of testosterone[74]. The metabolic clearance rate of androstenedione remains normal[74]. The result is an increase of the conversion of testosterone to androstenedione and, secondary, from androstenedione to estradiol. The second mechanism promoting the genesis of CHA seems to be an abnormal increase of the metabolization of estradiol to the less potent estriol[79]. The result is an inappropriate gonadotropin release[2] leading to CHA.

Treatment

The treatment of hypothyroidism consists in the substitution of thyroid function by the administration of pure thyroxine. Thyroxine has a half-life of about 7 days and is converted to the active triiodothyronine in the periphery. The daily amount of thyroid hormones needed is usually $100-175 \mu g$ thyroxine (T_4) per day orally. It is of utmost importance that, in frankly hypothyroid patients, the substitution should be started at a very low level and that the increase of the dosage should be done slowly.

Substitution by triiodothyronine (T_3) should be reserved for special indications. Fixed combinations of T_4 and T_3 are of no advantage and are nearly out of use.

Primary hypothyroidism is characterized by elevated basal values of TSH and by an exaggerated response to TRH. Secondary and tertiary hypothyroidism have extremely low basal values and no response to TRH. The monitoring of the substitution of primary hypothyroidism can be done by an ultrasensitive TSH assay or by the TRH test. In substituted patients, basal TSH and the TSH rise after TRH should lie within the normal range of healthy controls. In contrast, the substitution of pituitary or hypothalamic hypothyroidism cannot be monitored by basal TSH or by the TSH response to TRH. In these situations, the amount of T_4 needed has to be adjusted as a function of the clinic and of the serum levels of T_4 and of T_3.

OVARIAN HYPERTHECOSIS AND ANDROGEN-PRODUCING TUMORS

The term *ovarian hyperthecosis* was used for the first time by Fraenkel in 1943[80] to describe the theca interna hyperplasia of the ovary. Luteinization occurs frequently and has been accepted in the concept of hyperthecosis. Women with hyperthecosis are often described to be not only hirsute, but virilized, as shown by the presence of clitoromegaly. The definitive diagnosis has usually not been made until histology has been obtained by wedge resection or ovariectomy done for resistance to a conservative therapeutic approach. Following Yen, ovarian hyperthecosis has to be considered as a separate underlying disease for CHA. Yen enumerates five salient features which distinguish ovarian hyperthecosis from classical CHA[2]. However, there is an important clinical and pathological overlapping between ovarian hyperthecosis and classical CHA so that both conditions might be considered as different expressions of the same pathophysiological process[81-86]. Although failure to respond to induction of follicular maturation by clomiphene citrate has been reported to be characteristic for ovarian hyperthecosis[2], the same therapeutic principles have to be applied in patients suspected of hyperthecosis, as in classical CHA. Differential diagnosis with hilar cell hyperplasia or small hilar cell tumors of the ovary might be difficult[87,88].

Androgen-producing tumors of the ovary or of the adrenal[89-104] are extremely rare underlying diseases in CAH. The symptomatology of androgen-secreting tumors is not uniform, depending on the hormonal pattern produced. The prognosis is quite variable. The diagnostic approach comprises endocrine studies, computer-assisted tomography, magnetic resonance imaging and selective vein catheterization. Operative therapy with conservation of fertility is possible in some tumors, e.g. in androblastoma. In other, malignant, tumors, radical surgical extirpation, chemotherapy or radiotherapy have to be chosen depending on the tissular origin and the histological type.

CONCLUSIONS

Generally, underlying diseases responsible for chronic hyperandrogenic anovulation are characterized by an excessive or an insufficient production of, mostly, an extragonadal hormone. All these different extragonadal endocrine dysfunctions induce, by a common final pathophysiological step, an inappropriate gonadotropin secretion and an unfavorable intraovarian hyperandrogenic milieu, resulting in the clinical picture of chronic hyperandrogenic anovulation. In all these conditions, our therapeutical effort must concentrate on the correction of the underlying endocrinopathy. The treatment consists of the elimination or inhibition of an excessive hormone production or in the substitution of a missing endogenous hormone.

REFERENCES

1. Stein, I.F. and Leventhal, M.L. (1935). Amenorrhea associated with bilateral polycystic ovaries. *Am. J. Obstet. Gynecol.*, **29**, 181
2. Yen, S.S.C. (1980). The polycystic ovary syndrome. *Clin. Endocrinol.*, **12**, 177
3. Zumoff, B., Freeman, R., Coupey, S., Saenger, P., Markowitz, M. and Kream, J. (1983). A chronobiological abnormality in luteinizing hormone secretion in teenage girls with the polycystic ovary syndrome. *N. Engl. J. Med.*, **309**, 1206
4. Jones, G.E.S., Howard, J.E. and Langford, H. (1953). The use of cortisone in follicular phase disturbances. *Fertil. Steril.*, **4**, 49

5. White, P.C., New, M.I. and Dupont, B. (1987). Congenital adrenal hyperplasia. *N. Engl. J. Med.*, **316**, 1519 (part I), 1580 (part II)
6. New, M.I. and Speiser, P.W. (1986). Genetics of adrenal steroid 21-hydroxylase deficiency. *Endocr. Rev.*, **7**, 331
7. Dupont, B., Oberfield, S.E., Smithwick, E.M., Lee, T.D. and Levine, L.S. (1977). Close genetic linkage between HLA and congenital adrenal hyperplasia (21-hydroxylase deficiency). *Lancet*, **2**, 1309
8. Levine, L.S., Zachmann, M., New, M.I., Prader, A., Pollack, M.S., O'Neill, G.J., Pang, S.Y., Oberfield, S.E. and Dupont, B. (1978). Genetic mapping of the 21-hydroxylase deficiency gene within the HLA linkage group. *N. Engl. J. Med.*, **299**, 911
9. Kamilaris, T.C., DeBold, C.R., Manolas, K.J., Hoursanidis, A., Panageas, S. and Yiannatos, J. (1987). Testosterone-secreting adrenal adenoma in a peripubertal girl. *J. Am. Med. Assoc.*, **258**, 2558
10. Abraham, G.E. (1974). Ovarian and adrenal contribution to peripheral androgens during the menstrual cycle. *J. Clin. Endocrinol. Metab.*, **39**, 340
11. Kohn, B., Levine, L.S., Pollack, M.S., Pang, S., Lorenzen, F., Levy, D.J., Lerner, A.J., Gian, F.R., Dupont, B. and New, M.I. (1982). Late-onset steroid 21-hydroxylase deficiency: a variant of classical congenital adrenal hyperplasia. *J. Clin. Endocrinol. Metab.*, **55**, 817
12. Brodie, B.L. and Wentz, A.C. (1987). Late onset congenital adrenal hyperplasia: a gynecologist's perspective. *Fertil. Steril.*, **48**, 175
13. Lee, P.A., Rosenwaks, Z., Urban, D.M., Migeon, C.J. and Bias, W. (1982). Attenuated forms of congenital adrenal hyperplasia due to 21-hydroxylase deficiency. *J. Clin. Endocrinol. Metab.*, **55**, 866
14. New, M.I., Dupont, B., Pollack, M.S. and Levine, L.S. (1981). The biochemical basis for genotyping 21-hydroxylase deficiency. *Hum. Genet.*, **58**, 123
15. Bongiovanni, A.M. (1986). Late-onset adrenal hyperplasia (letter). *N. Engl. J. Med.*, **314**, 450
16. Rosenfield, R.L., Rich, B.H., Wolfsdorf, J.L., Cassorla, F., Parks, J.S., Bongiovanni, A.M., Wu, C.H. and Shackleton, C.H.L. (1980). Pubertal presentation of congenital 5-3β-hydroxysteroid dehydrogenase deficiency. *J. Clin. Endocrinol. Metab.*, **51**, 345
17. Pang, S., Lerner, A.J., Stoner, E., Levine, L.S., Oberfield, S.E., Engel, I. and New, M.I. (1985). Late-onset adrenal steroid 3β-hydroxysteroid dehydrogenase deficiency. I. A case of hirsutism in pubertal and post-pubertal women. *J. Clin. Endocrinol. Metab.*, **60**, 428
18. Lobo, R.A. and Goebelsmann, U. (1981). Evidence for reduced 3β-ol-hydroxysteroid dehydrogenase activity in some hirsute women thought to have polycystic ovarian syndrome. *J. Clin. Endocrinol. Metab.*, **53**, 394
19. Bongiovanni, A.M. (1984). Congenital adrenal hyperplasia due to 3β-hydroxysteroid dehydrogenase deficiency. In New, M.I. and Levine, L.S. (eds.) *Adrenal Diseases in Childhood*, Vol. 13, p. 72. (New York: S. Karger)
20. Boyers, S.P., Buster, J.E. and Marshall, J.R. (1982). Hypothalamic–pituitary–adrenocortical function during long-term low-dose dexamethasone therapy in hyperandrogenized women. *Am. J. Obstet. Gynecol.*, **142**, 330
21. Speiser, P.W., Dupont, B., Rubenstein, P., Piazza, A., Kastelan, A. and New, M.I. (1985). High frequency of non-classical steroid 21-hydroxylase deficiency. *Am. J. Hum. Genet.*, **37** 650
22. Chrousos, G.P., Evans, M.I., Loriaux, L.D., McCluskey, J., Fletcher, J.C. and Schulman, J.D. (1985). Prenatal therapy in congenital adrenal hyperplasia. *Ann. N.Y. Acad. Sci.*, **458**, 156
23. Chrousos, G.P., Loriaux, L.D., Mann, D.L. and Cutler, G.B. (1982). Late-onset 21-hydroxylase deficiency mimicking idiopathic hirsutism or polycystic ovarian disease: an allelic variant of congenital virilizing adrenal hyperplasia with a milder enzymatic defect. *Ann. Intern. Med.*, **96**, 143
24. Emans, S.J., Grace, E., Fleishnick, E., Mansfield, M.J. and Crigler, J.F. Jr. (1983). Detection of late-onset 21-hydroxylase deficiency congenital adrenal hyperplasia in adolescents. *Pediatrics*, **72**, 690
25. Lobo, R.A. and Goebelsmann, U. (1980). Adult manifestation of congenital adrenal hyperplasia due to incomplete 21-hydroxylase deficiency mimicking polycystic ovarian disease. *Am. J. Obstet. Gynecol.*, **138**, 720

26. Carmina, E., Gagliano, A.M., Rosato, F., Maggiore, M. and Janni, A. (1984). The endocrine pattern of late onset adrenal hyperplasias (21-hydroxylase deficiency). *J. Endocrinol. Invest.*, **7**, 89

27. Benjamin, F., Deutsch, S., Saperstein, H. and Seltzer, V. (1986). Prevalence of and markers for the attenuated form of congenital adrenal hyperplasia and hyperprolactinemia masquerading as polycystic ovarian disease. *Fertil. Steril.*, **46**, 215

28. Chetkowski, R.J., DeFazio, J., Shamonki, I., Judd, H.L. and Chang, J. (1984). The incidence of late-onset congenital adrenal hyperplasia due to 21-hydroxylase deficiency among hirsute women. *J. Clin. Endocrinol. Metab.*, **58**, 595

29. New, M.I., Lorenzen, F., Lerner, A.J., Kohn, B., Oberfield, S.E., Pollack, M.S., Dupont, B., Stoner, E., Levy, D.J., Pang, S. and Levine, L. (1983). Genotyping steroid 21-hydroxylase deficiency: hormonal reference data. *J. Clin. Endocrinol. Metab.*, **57**, 320

30. Ferriman, D., Purdie, A.W. and Tindall, W.J. (1961). The use of corticosteroids in infertility associated with hirsutism and oligomenorrhea. *Br. Med. J.*, **1**, 1006

31. Sarris, S., Swyer, G.I.M., Ward, R.H.T., Lawrence, D.M. and McGarrigle, H.H. (1978). The treatment of mild adrenal hyperplasia and associated infertility with prednisone. *Br. J. Obstet. Gynaecol.*, **85**, 251

32. Blankenstein, J., Faiman, C., Reyes, F.I., Schroeder, M.L. and Winter, J.S.D. (1980). Adult-onset familial adrenal 21-hydroxylase deficiency. *Am. J. Med.*, **68**, 441

33. Birnbaum, M.D. and Rose, L.I. (1984). Late onset adrenocortical hydroxylase deficiencies associated with menstrual dysfunction. *Obstet. Gynecol.*, **63**, 445

34. Maroulis, G.B. (1981). Evaluation of hirsutism and hyperandrogenemia. *Fertil. Steril.*, **36**, 273

35. Mahesh, V.B., Greenblatt, R.B. and Coniff, R.F. (1968). Adrenal hyperplasia: a case report of delayed onset of the congenital form or an acquired form. *J. Clin. Endocrinol. Metab.*, **28**, 619

36. Steinberger, E., Smith, D.K., Tcholakian, R.K. and Rodriguez-Rigau, L.J. (1979). Testosterone levels in female partners of infertile couples. *Am. J. Obstet. Gynecol.*, **133**, 133

37. Raj, S.G., Thompson, I.E., Berger, M.J. and Taymor, M.L. (1977). Clinical aspects of the polycystic ovary syndrome. *Obstet. Gynecol.*, **49**, 552

38. Zarate, A., Hernandez-Ayup, S. and Rios-Montiel, A. (1971). Treatment of anovulation in the Stein–Leventhal syndrome. Analysis of 90 cases. *Fertil. Steril.*, **221**, 188

39. Rodriguez-Rigau, L.J., Smith, K.D., Tcholakian, R.K. and Steinberger, E. (1979). Effect of prednisone on plasma testosterone levels and on duration of phases of the menstrual cycle in hyperandrogenic women. *Fertil. Steril.*, **32**, 408

40. Smith, D.K., Rodriguez-Rigau, L.J., Tcholakian, R.K. and Steinberger, E. (1979). The relation between plasma testosterone levels and the lengths of phases of the menstrual cycle. *Fertil. Steril.*, **32**, 403

41. Smith, D.K., Steinberger, E. and Perloff, W.H. (1965). Polycystic ovarian disease. A report of 301 patients. *Am. J. Obstet. Gynecol.*, **93**, 994

42. Toaff, R., Toaff, M.E., Gould, S. and Chayen, R. (1978). Role of androgenic hyperactivity in anovulation. *Fertil. Steril.*, **29**, 407

43. Kirscher, M.A., Zucker, I.R. and Jespersen, D. (1976). Idiopathic hirsutism. An ovarian abnormality. *N. Engl. J. Med.*, **294**, 637

44. Maroulis, G.B. (1981). Evaluation of hirsutism and hyperandrogenemia. *Fertil. Steril.*, **36**, 273

45. Maroulis, G.B. (1984). Polycystic ovarian disease and dexamethasone. *Semin. Reprod. Endocrinol.*, **2**, 263

46. Rittmaster, R., Loriaux, D.L. and Cutler, G.B. Jr. (1985) Sensitivity of cortisol and adrenal androgens to dexamethasone suppression in hirsute women. *J. Clin. Endocrinol. Metab.*, **61**, 462

47. Wentz, A.C. Gutai, J.P., Jones, G.S. and Migeon, C.J. (1976). Ovarian hyperthecosis in the adolescent patient. *J. Pediatr.*, **88**, 488–93

48. Steinberger, E., Smith, K.D. and Rodriguez-Rigau, L.J. (1981). Hyperandrogenism and female infertility. In Crosignani, P.G. and Rubin, B.L. (eds.) *Endocrinology of Human Infertility: New Aspects*, pp. 327–34. (London: Academic Press)

49. Madden, J.D., Milewich, L. and Gomez-Sanchez, C. (1977). The effect of oral contraceptive treatment on the serum concentration of dehydroepiandrosterone sulfate and ACTH.

Gynecol. Invest., **8**, 16

50. Madden, J.D., Milewich, L., Parker, C.R., Carr, B.R., Boyar, R.M. and MacDonald, P.C. (1978). The effect of oral contraceptive treatment on the serum concentration of dehydroepiandrosterone sulfate. *Am. J. Obstet. Gynecol.*, **132**, 380

51. Symington, T.S. (1969). *The Functional Pathology of the Human Adrenal Gland.* (Edinburgh, London: E. &. S. Livingston)

52. Burke, C.W. and Beardwell, G.G. (1972). Cushing's syndrome. *Q. J. Med.*, **42**, 175

53. Ross, E.J., Marshall-Jones, P. and Friedman, M. (1966). Cushing's syndrome: diagnostic criteria. *Q. J. Med.*, **35**, 149

54. Hogan, T.F., Gilchrist, K.W., Westring, D.W. and Citrin, D. L. (1980). A clinical and pathological study of adrenocortical carcinoma: therapeutic implications. *Cancer*, **45**, 2880

55. Soffer, L.J., Dorfmann, R.J. and Gabrilove, J.L. (1961). *The Human Adrenal Gland.* (Philadelphia: Lea & Febiger)

56. Ross, E.J. and Linch, D.C. (1982). Cushing's syndrome – killing disease. Discriminatory values of signs and symptoms aiding early diagnosis. *Lancet*, **2**, 646

57. Flury, A., Müller, J., Froesch, E.R. and Labhart, A. (1971). Das Cushing-Syndrom. Kasuistische Zusammenstellung von 43 Cushing-Patienten der Medizinischen Univ.-Klinik Zürich von 1958–1969. *Schweiz Med. Wochenschr.*, **101**, 313

58. Rees, L.H. and Landon, J. (1976). Biochemical abnormalities in some human neoplasms: inappropriate biosynthesis of hormones by tumors. In Symington, T.S. and Carter, R.L. (eds.) *Scientific Foundation of Oncology*, p. 112 (London: Heinemann Medical Books)

59. Chrousos, G.P., Schulte, H.M., Oldfield, E.H., Gold, P.W., Cutler, G.B. and Loriaux, D.L. (1984). The corticotropin-releasing-factor stimulation test: an aid in the evaluation of patients with Cushing's syndrome. *N. Engl. J. Med.*, **310**, 622

60. Burch, W. (1983). A survey of results with transsphenoidal surgery in Cushing's disease. *N. Engl. J. Med.*, **308**, 103

61. Kelly, W.F., MacFarlane, I.A., Longson, D., Davies, D. and Sutcliffe, H. (1983). Cushing's disease treated by total adrenalectomy: long-term observations of 43 patients. *Q. J. Med.*, **52**, 224

62. Cassar, J., Doyle, F.H., Lewis, P.D., Mashiter, K., Van Noorden, S. and Joplin, G.F. (1976). Treatment of Nelson's syndrome by pituitary implantation of yttrium-90 or gold 198. *Br. Med. J.*, **2**, 269

63. Luton, J.P., Mahoudeau, J.A., Bouchard, Ph., Thieblot, Ph. Hautecouverture, M., Simon, D., Laudat, M.H., Touitou, U. and Bricaire, H. (1979). Treatment of Cushing's disease by o,p'DDD, survey of 62 cases. *N. Engl. J. Med.*, **300**, 459

64. Schteingart, D.E., Tsao, H.S., Taylor, Ch.I., McKenzie, A., Victoria, R. and Therrien, B.A. (1980). Sustained remission of Cushing's disease with mitotane and pituitary irradiation. *Ann. Intern. Med.*, **92**, 613

65. Orth, D.N. (1984). The old and the new in Cushing's syndrome. *N. Engl. J. Med.*, **310**, 649

66. Cooper, P.R. and Shucart, W.M. (1979). Treatment of Cushing's disease with o,p'-DDD. *N. Engl. J. Med.*, **301**, 48

67. Bricaire, H., Luton, J.P. and Mahoudeau, J.A. (1979). Treatment of Cushing's disease with o,p'-DDD. *N. Engl. J. Med.*, **301**, 49

68. Orth, D.N. and Liddle, G.W. (1971). Results of treatment in 108 patients with Cushing's syndrome. *N. Engl. J. Med.*, **285**, 243

69. Santen, R.J., Samojlik, E., Lipton, A., Harvey, H., Ruby, E.B., Wells, S.A. and Kendall, J. (1977). Kinetic hormonal and clinical studies with aminoglutethimide in breast cancer. *Cancer*, **39**, 2948

70. Child, D.F., Burke, C.W., Burley, D.M., Rees, L.H. and Fraser, T.R. (1976). Drug control of Cushing's syndrome. Combined aminoglutethimide and metyrapone therapy. *Acta Endocrinol.*, **82**, 330

71. Angeli, A. and Frairia, R. (1985). Ketoconazole therapy in Cushing's disease. *Lancet*, **1**, 821

72. Conteras, P., Rojas, A., Biagini, L., Gonzales, P. and Massardo, T. (1985). Regression of metastatic adrenal carcinoma during palliative ketoconazole treatment. *Lancet*, **2**, 151

73. Sheperd, F.A., Hoffert, B., Evans, W.K., Emery, G. and Trachtenberg, J. (1985). Ketoconazole: use in the treatment of ectopic adrenocorticotropic hormone production and Cushing's syndrome in small-cell lung cancer. *Arch. Intern. Med.*, **145**, 863

74. Gordon, G.G., Southren, A.L., Tochimoto, S., Rand, J.J. and Olivo, J. (1969). Effect of hyperthyroidism and hypothyroidism on the metabolism of testosterone and androstenedione in man. *J. Clin. Endocrinol. Metab.*, **29**, 164

75. Ruder, H., Carvol, P., Mahoudeau, J.A., Ross, G.T. and Lipsett, M.B. (1971). Effects of induced hyperthyroidism on steroid metabolism in man. *J. Clin. Endocrinol. Metab.*, **33**, 382

76. Southren, A.I., Olivo, J., Gordon, G.G., Vittek, J., Brener, J. and Fafii, F. (1974). The conversion of androgens to estrogens in hyperthyroidism. *J. Clin. Endocrinol. Metab.*, **38**, 207

77. Chopra, I.J. and Tulchinsky, D. (1974). Status of estrogen–androgen balance in hyperthyroid men with Grave's disease. *J. Clin. Endocrinol. Metab.*, **38**, 269

78. Fishman, J., Hellman, L., Zumoff, B. and Gallagher, T.F. (1965). Effect of thyroid on hydroxylation of estrogen in man. *J. Clin. Endocrinol. Metab.*, **25**, 365

79. Fishman, J., Hellman, L. and Zumoff, B. (1962). Influence of thyroid hormone on estrogen metabolism in man. *J. Clin. Endocrinol. Metab.*, **22**, 389

80. Fraenkel, L. (1943). Thecoma and hyperthecosis of the ovary. *J. Clin. Endocrinol. Metab.*, **3**, 557

81. Aiman, J., Edman, C.D., Worley, R.J., Vellios, F. and MacDonald, P.C. (1978). Androgen and estrogen formation in women with ovarian hyperthecosis. *Obstet. Gynecol.*, **51**, 1

82. Givens, J.R., Wiser, W.L., Coleman, S.A., Wilroy, R.S., Andersen, R.N. and Fish, S.A. (1971). Familial ovarian hyperthecosis. A study of two families. *Am. J. Obstet. Gynecol.*, **110**, 959

83. Sohval, A.R. (1956). Diseases of the ovary. In Soffer, L.J. (ed.) *Diseases of the Endocrine Glands*, 2nd edn., pp. 664–741. (Philadelphia: Lea & Febiger)

84. Case records of the Massachusetts General Hospital (Case 12-1974). (1974). *N. Engl. J. Med.*, **290**, 730

85. Aiman, J., Nalick, R.H., Jacobs, A., Porter, J.C., Edman, C.D., Vellios, F. and MacDonald, P.C. (1977). The origin of androgen and estrogen in a virilized postmenopausal woman with bilateral cystic teratomas. *Obstet. Gynecol.*, **49**, 695

86. Sommers, S. C. and Wadman, P.J. (1956). Pathogenesis of polycystic ovaries. *Am. J. Obstet. Gynecol.*, **72**, 160

87. Bardin, C.W., Lipsett, M.B., Edgcomb, J.H. and Marshall, J.R. (1967). Studies of testosterone metabolism in a patient with masculinization due to stromal hyperthecosis. *N. Engl. J. Med.*, **277**, 399

88. Steinberg, W.H. (1949). The morphology, androgenic function, hyperplasia and tumors of the ovarian hilus cells. *Am. J. Pathol.*, **25**, 493

89. Birkhäuser, M.H. (1989). Endokrin aktive Genitaltumoren. *Therapeutische Umschau*, **46**, 895

90. Bertagna, C. and Orth, D.N. (1981). Clinical and laboratory findings and results of therapy in 58 patients with adrenocortical tumors admitted to a single medical center (1951 to 1978). *Am. J. Med.*, **71**, 855

91. Casthely, S., Diamandis, H.P. and Pierre-Louis, R. (1977). Hilar cell tumor of the ovary: diagnostic value of plasma testosterone by selective ovarian vein catheterization. *Am. J. Obstet. Gynecol.*, **129**, 108

92. Evans, A.T. III., Gaffey, T.A., Malkasian, G.D. Jr. and Annegers, J. F. (1980). Clinicopathologic review of 118 granulosa and 82 theca cell tumors. *Obstet. Gynecol.*, **55**, 231

93. Gabrilove, J.L., Seman, A.T., Sabet, R., Mitty, H.A. and Nicolis, G.L. (1981). Virilizing adrenal adenoma with studies on the steroid content of the adrenal venous effluent and a review of the literature. *Endocr. Rev.*, **2**, 462

94. Ireland, K. and Woodruff, J.D., (1976). Masculinizing ovarian tumors. *Obstet. Gynecol. Surv.*, **31**, 83

95. Jones, H.W. Jr. (1976). Editorial comment. *Obstet. Gynecol. Surv.*, **31**, 217

96. Kable, W.T. and Yussmann, M.A. (1979). Testosterone-secreting adrenal adenoma. *Fertil. Steril.*, **32**, 610

97. Scully, R.E. (1977). Ovarian tumors. A review. *Am. J. Pathol.*, **87**, 686

98. Serov, S.F., Scully, R.E. and Sobin, L.H. (1973). Histological typing of ovarian tumors. *Int. Histol. Classif. Tumors*, 9, WHO, Geneva

99. Sternberg, W.H. and Dhurander, H.N. (1977). Functional ovarian tumors of stromal and

sex cord origin. *Human Pathol.*, **8**, 565

100. Sternberg, W.H. and Roth, L.M. (1973). Ovarian stromal tumors containing Leydig cells. I., Stromal Leydig cell tumor and non-neoplastic transformation of ovarian stroma to Leydig cells. *Cancer*, **32**, 940

101. Tavassoli, F.A. and Norris, H.J. (1980). Sertoli cell tumors of the ovary,. A clinico-pathological study of 28 cases with ultrastructural observations. *Cancer*, **46**, 2281

102. Weiland, A.J., Bookstein, J.J., Clearly, R.E. and Judd, H.L. (1978). Preoperative localization of virilizing tumors by selective venous sampling. *Am. J. Obstet. Gynecol.*, **131**, 797

103. Wentz, A.C., White, R.I. Jr., Migeon, C.J., Hsu, T.H., Barnes, H.V. and Jones, G.S. (1976). Differential ovarian and adrenal vein catheterization. *Am. J. Obstet. Gynecol.*, **125**, 1000

104. Werk, E.E., Sholiton, L.J. and Kalejs, L. (1973). Testosterone-secreting adrenal adenoma under gonadotropin control. *N. Engl. J. Med.*, **289**, 767

9

Hormonal response of polycystic ovaries to administration of clomiphene citrate

R.E. Lappöhn

Approximately one-third of all fertility disturbances is caused by anovulation. Then, in the absence of ovarian failure, induction of ovulation is the most successful of all infertility treatments. Even though, 25 years after its introduction, its method of action is uncertain, clomiphene is the initial treatment of choice in most instances. Even if started empirically, many patients conceive within three treatment courses. However, from the outset people have been wondering about the discrepancy between the number of apparently ovulatory reactions and the number of conceptions.

Our early results prompted the question whether a common basic disturbance of ovarian function, be it anatomic or functional, and possibly related to obesity and hirsutism, prevented conception in apparently ovulating women. In the period when radioimmunoassays first came into use, a prospective study was started[1]. Sixteen clomiphene-induced cycles which resulted in conception were followed, with daily determinations of pregnanediol and pregnanetriol excretions in early morning urine and determinations of serum gonadotropins and estradiol in the highest possible frequency. They were compared to the results obtained in six women with proven fertility. In non-obese women without hirsutism, the results were not significantly different from those obtained in normal women. Ten conceptions occurred in obese and/or hirsute patients, after total dosages of between 500 and 1250 mg clomiphene citrate (median 700). There were four abortions and six normal pregnancies. The only differences with the reference cycles were a somewhat higher pregnanetriol excretion in both phases of the cycle and high luteinizing hormone (LH) values in the follicular phase of four cycles. Basal luteinizing hormone/follicle stimulating hormone (LH/FSH) ratios were > 3 in five patients with a successful pregnancy and in all cycles ending in abortion.

In contrast, apparently ovulatory cycles in seven women with obesity and/or hirsutism who did not conceive were characterized by:

(1) A lower than normal excretion of pregnanediol in the luteal phase;

(2) Low or low–normal estradiol in the follicular phase, but normal levels in the luteal phase;

(3) Slightly elevated pregnanetriol values throughout the cycle. Similarly to conception cycles, pregnanetriol excretion remained elevated in women who also received prednisone;

(4) Follicular phase LH rose to high levels in most women, but FSH was unremarkable.

Low values for progesterone/pregnanediol in the luteal phase of the cycle are known as luteal insufficiency, as described by Sherman and Korenman in spontaneous cycles from obese women[2]. In their report follicular phase estradiol values were normal. Most of our clomiphene-induced cycles showed a low follicular phase estradiol. An accepted explanation for luteal insufficiency is that it is caused by defective granulosa cell function in the follicular phase of the cycle. FSH levels were normal in most of these patients and therefore an absolute shortage of FSH is unlikely as an explanation of the defective granulosa cell function. Good possibilities are a *relative* shortage of FSH or a follicular insensitivity to its action. Either an absolute or a relative shortage of FSH may lead to increased atresia, a phenomenon that is also related to relative hyperstimulation by LH and to LH-dependent hyperandrogenism. Of course, degenerated granulosa cells are unable to respond adequately to a FSH stimulus.

The elevated excretion of pregnanetriol was unexplicable at the time; adrenal and ovarian sources of 17-hydroxyprogesterone were both possible. In many of these patients, reduction of circulating androgens by suppressing the adrenal contribution at night and also successful dieting or the use of higher doses of clomiphene citrate led to pregnancy. Treatment with human menopausal gonadotropin or chorionic gonadotropin (hMG/CG) was not successful: 11 courses in seven patients who did not ovulate after clomiphene citrate led to one normal pregnancy. More or less as a last resort bilateral ovarian wedge resection was performed in six of these patients and all became pregnant within a year after the operation.

The long-term fertility of patients who had a bilateral ovarian wedge resection has recently been described[3]. In short, patients with polycystic ovaries and hyperplastic stromal abnormalities (stroma hyperplasia, hyperthecosis and small thecomas) had most spontaneous conceptions and a normal fertility during long-term follow-up; women with polycystic ovaries without stromal abnormalities also had a normal long-term fecundability, but more often needed postoperative stimulation of ovulation in order to conceive. Finally, women with large ovaries, histologically normal stroma and small follicles, as well as those with large follicles and cysts without theca cell activity, did not benefit from surgery. It is of interest that, with the exception of the women with very large ovaries and small follicles, who as a group had a lower LH/FSH ratio, all women had identical basal hormone values.

From about 1980, after exclusion of male infertility, hyperprolactinemia, metabolic disease and serious psychological disturbances/psychiatric disease, a clomiphene test has been used as the corner stone of our diagnostic procedure. In women with an elevated LH/FSH ratio and/or clinical or biochemical hyperandrogenism, clomiphene citrate, 100 mg from day 4 to day 8, is prescribed. If necessary, withdrawal bleeding is induced with medroxyprogesterone acetate, 10 mg daily for 10 days. Presently, vaginal echoscopy is used to monitor the ovarian response, but ultrasound examinations were started with a compound grey scale B scan, to be replaced by a real-time abdominal sector scan in 1981. Since with that technique only follicles over 0.8 cm can be identified, echoscopy was started at day 10 and repeated every third day.

In our hands, abdominal ultrasound proved to be of little value in distinguishing women with polycystic ovaries with stromal abnormalities from those without; echodense stromal areas were mainly found to correlate with the presence of corpora albicantia and it was impossible to quantify the amount of stromal tissue. On the other hand, using the criteria given by Adams et al.[4], those not having polycystic ovaries could be recognized in retrospect. The different prognosis of the bilateral ovarian wedge resection between women with and without stromal abnormalities still makes a differentiation useful; the question arose whether there would be a different hormonal response in the clomiphene test.

Estradiol, total testosterone, androstenedione, 17-hydroxyprogesterone and dehydroepiandrosterone sulfate (DHEAS) in selected cases (elevated for age) were determined by radioimmunoassay in samples obtained at days 4 and 8 and each day of echoscopy. The latter was performed twice in the presumably luteal phase of the cycle, 3 and 7 days after the largest follicle had disappeared, collapsed or reached a diameter of at least 1.8 cm. Progesterone was determined at the last three ultrasound examinations. Blood samples were generally taken about noon.

In order to find out whether patients with histologically proven polycystic ovary syndrome with and without stromal abnormalities have different hormonal reactions in the clomiphene test, the results of normal clomiphene-induced cycles (four of which occurred with conception) from women with hyperandrogenic anovulation were compared with 23 test cycles of those who later underwent a bilateral ovarian wedge resection. The estradiol and progesterone results of the clomiphene-induced normal cycles include those of women with basal DHEAS levels $> 8 \mu$mol/l, who received dexamethasone, 0.5 mg at 11p.m.

There were 12 anovulatory clomiphene citrate tests; five occurred in women who later proved to have stromal disease (hyperthecosis, small thecomas); in five others the ovaries were greatly enlarged and had a thick tunica, but otherwise had not enough characteristics of polycystic ovary syndrome. Two women were grossly obese, and also had insufficient histological characteristics for a diagnosis of polycystic ovary syndrome. Estradiol rose over 0.8 nmol/l in only one cycle; a dominant follicle was seen. All other patients showed the development of many, often more than 20, small follicles never growing larger than 1 cm. The initial estradiol increase in these cycles was normal and there were no differences between cycles in patients with and without stromal disease. Androstenedione, testosterone and 17-hydroxyprogesterone all increased in the course of the test; the increase of testosterone from day 4 to day 8 in patients with stromal disease was significantly higher than in those without; otherwise there were no differences.

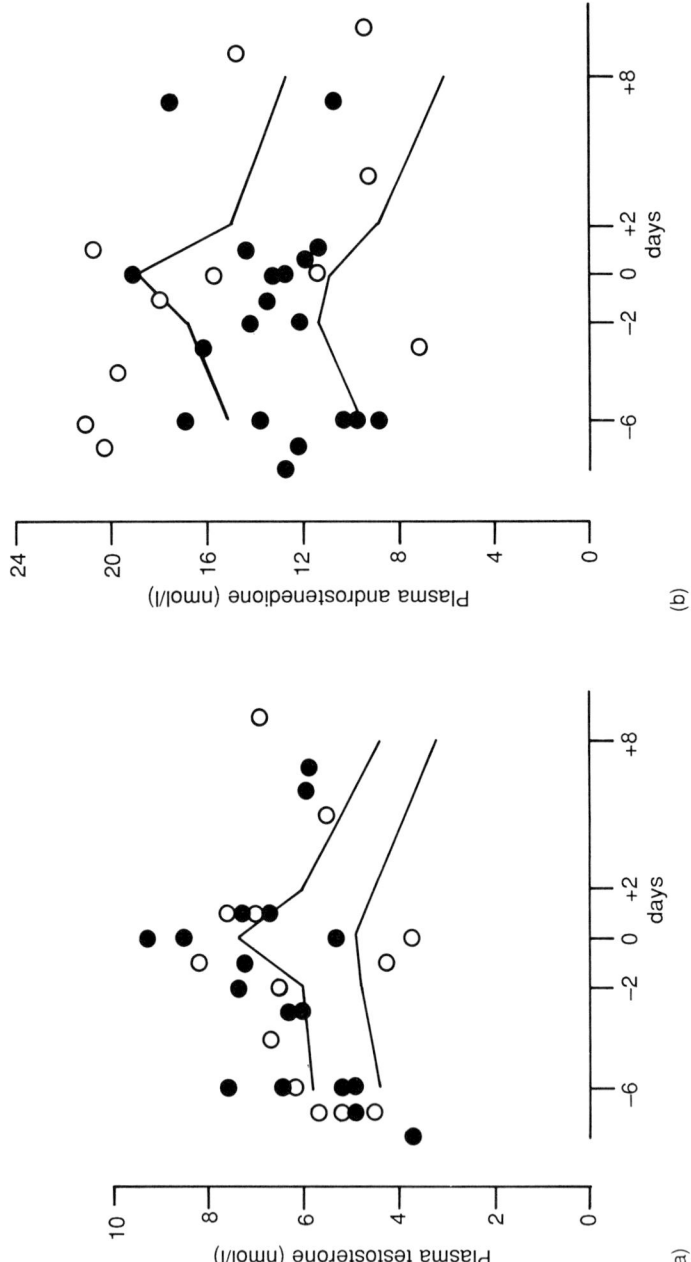

Figure 1 Clomiphene test before bilateral ovarian wedge resection. (a) Plasma testosterone levels; (b) plasma androstenedione levels in cycles with approximately normal luteal progesterone levels in five women with normal (open circles) and seven with pathological (closed circles) ovarian stroma

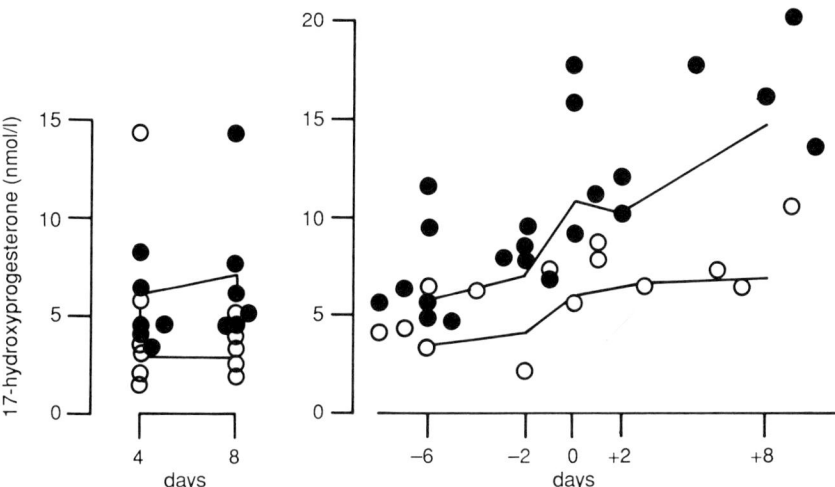

Figure 2 Clomiphene test before bilateral ovarian wedge resection. 17-Hydroxyprogesterone levels in cycles with approximately normal luteal progesterone levels in five women with normal (open circles) and seven with pathological (closed circles) ovarian stroma

In 12 cycles with progesterone production, the results for estradiol and progesterone were comparable to the earlier findings. Five of these cycles occurred in women with polycystic ovary syndrome and stroma hyperplasia, two in women with polycystic ovaries and hyperthecosis and five in women with polycystic ovaries without stromal abnormalities. Again, there was a sharp increase of plasma androgens in the course of the follicular phase. In the women with stromal disease, the increase of testosterone was higher than in those without (Figure 1a). The androstenedione response in women without stromal abnormalities at first glance was higher than in women with stromal hyperplasia and hyperthecosis (Figure 1b) and testosterone seemed to be higher in the latter, but the differences were not significant. Throughout the cycle, however, the 17-hydroxyprogesterone concentrations in the women with stromal disorders were higher (Figure 2). With the exception of two cycles, one bifollicular, ultrasound examination failed to show normal follicular growth until 20 mm and follicular collapse. Multiple follicle growth was present in all cases, and filling in of the dominant follicle occurred at the time of the LH peak or the increase of plasma progesterone.

In the same way as in women with insufficient gonadotropic stimulation of ovarian activity, clomiphene citrate can stimulate follicular maturation and ovulation in women with hyperandrogenic anovulation. Since, in cycles with conception, normal values of follicular estradiol and luteal progesterone are found simultaneously with elevated androgens and hydroxyprogesterone, the former are the product of the growing dominant follicle, and the latter probably arise from unhealthy follicles, atretic ones and the ovarian stroma. The increased ovarian production of testosterone may, especially in its reduced form, contribute to atresia of the small antral follicles. The role of 17α-hydroxyprogesterone in this respect is unclear. At one time, it was considered as an early indicator of follicular luteinization[5]. It is a product of the theca cells[6] and may, if present in relatively high concentration, merely indicate an overflow of substrate to the C17–21 lyase (desmolase) system. Normally this system at the beginning of the LH peak is inhibited by the high (pre-ovulatory) levels of estradiol and its inhibition results in a less effective production of androgens and estradiol. Under the circumstances considered above, however, it may be a sign of hyperstimulation of the ovary by LH. It may identify the patients who, failing treatment with clomiphene citrate, benefit from surgical treatment of their chronic anovulation.

REFERENCES

1. Lappöhn, R.E. (1977). Stoornissen in de follikelrijping bij ovulatie-inductie met clomipheen. *Thesis*, Groningen
2. Sherman, B.M. and Korenman, S.G. (1974). Measurement of serum LH, FSH, estradiol and progesterone in disorders of the human menstrual cycle: the inadequate luteal phase. *J. Clin. Metab. Endocrinol.*, **39**, 145
3. Lappöhn, R.E. and Bogchelman, D.H. (1989). The relation of fertility and ovarian histology after bilateral ovarian wedge resection. *Fertil. Steril.*, **52**, 221
4. Adams, J., Polson, D.W. and Franks, S. (1986). Prevalence of polycystic ovaries in women with anovulation and idiopathic hirsutism. *Br. Med. J.*, **293**, 355–9
5. Thorneycroft, I.H., Mishell, D., Stone, S.C. *et al.* (1971). The relation of serum 17-hydroxyprogesterone and estradiol-17β levels during the human menstrual cycle. *Am. J. Obstet. Gynecol.*, **111**, 947
6. Channing, C.P. (1969). The production of 17α-hydroxyprogesterone in porcine ovarian theca cells. *J. Endocrinol.*, **45**, 297

10

Induction of ovulation with human gonadotropins

M. Breckwoldt and H.P. Zahradnik

INTRODUCTION

Exogenous administration of human gonadotropins is the most powerful therapeutic regimen to stimulate ovarian function. Follicular maturation can be achieved by the use of either pituitary gonadotropins or gonadotropins extracted from postmenopausal urine. For the induction of ovulation with the release of a mature ovum the additional administration of human chorionic gonadotropin (hCG) is required. The first pregnancy achieved by this therapeutic approach was reported by Gemzell in 1960[1]. Primarily, human pituitary extracts were used for the induction of follicular development in amenorrheic infertile patients[1-3]. Almost simultaneously, human menopausal gonadotropins (hMG) came into clinical use[4]. Despite the differences in chemistry and biological activity, pituitary and urinary preparations proved to be equally effective in terms of clinical response[3]. Since postmortem pituitaries are in limited supply today, only hMG preparations are used for stimulation of ovarian function in patients whose sterility is due to chronic anovulation.

hMG/hCG treatment can be associated with severe complications such as ovarian hyperstimulation, multiple ovulation and, consequently, multiple births. Therefore several preconditions and precautions have to be considered, namely selection of patients, treatment schedule, and treatment monitoring.

SELECTION OF PATIENTS

Based on the classification proposed by the WHO, there are only two major groups of patients who can be considered candidates for hMG/hCG therapy, in particular those with low gonadotropin levels and low or undetectable estrogen production. The prolactin levels in these patients are in the lower normal range. In these patients, classified as group I, gonadotropin therapy is highly effective in achieving pregnancy rates of the order of 80%[5].

In anovulatory patients with normal gonadotropin levels and detectable estrogen production, also referred to as WHO group II, clomiphene is the first treatment of choice for induction of ovulation. If, however, these patients fail to respond to clomiphene treatment, hMG/hCG therapy is indicated. This group of patients, which also includes patients with polycystic ovary syndrome, is difficult to treat, pregnancy rates are low, and the incidence of complications is rather high. Ovarian hyperstimulation is frequently observed, and premature luteinizing hormone (LH) surges and subsequent luteinization complicate the treatment course. Premature LH surges are probably due to the presence of endogenous LH and follicle stimulating hormone (FSH) stored in the pituitary being readily released by the rising estrogen levels, inducing a positive feedback reaction. The premature LH output can be reliably avoided by pretreatment with gonadotropin releasing hormone (GnRH) agonists, as shown in many clinical studies. This regimen, however, does not eliminate the risk of ovarian hyperstimulation[6].

TREATMENT SCHEDULE

Various proposals have been made for the use of human gonadotropins in patients with chronic anovulatory infertility. However, there is general agreement that the individually adjusted dosage of hMG, according to the ovarian response, is the most meaningful approach. This recommendation is outlined in Figure 1, indicating that the treatment course starts with a low dose of 1–2 ampules of hMG daily for 5–6 days. If this dose is below the threshold of ovarian sensitivity, the dose should be increased by 1 ampule per day. Having reached the effective dose, the hMG administration is kept constant until the leading follicle has reached its optimal size for ovulation induction.

Ovarian response is monitored daily during the active phase. Ovarian estrogen secretion is easily recognized by vaginal cytology and cervical parameters, such as Spinnbarkeit and ferning of the cervical mucus. Insler has proposed a score to semiquantitate estrogen production[7]. More reliable data, however, are obtained from estrogen determinations in 24 h urine samples or in serum. Serum estradiol levels of 500–1200 pg/ml, associated with the presence of one or two dominant follicles with a diameter of 17–20 mm, indicate optimal conditions for the administration of hCG. During recent years, ultrasonography with vaginal scanning and high resolution has become increasingly important in monitoring ovarian function. This technique allows direct visualization of the growing follicles. Growth velocity, number of follicles and their shape can all be observed. This technique is extremely helpful in timing the application of hCG for ovulation induction. In addition, the risk of ovarian hyperstimulation can be predicted, and the administration of hCG can be withheld.

During exogenous hMG administration, all physiological mechanisms that normally regulate ovarian function and ultimately guarantee mono-ovulation are overruled. Therefore hMG treatment must be regarded as a pharmacological approach to ovarian dysfunction; ovarian hyperstimulation is in most cases of no clinical relevance. However, endocrine parameters such as urinary estrogen output or plasma levels of estrogens and pro-

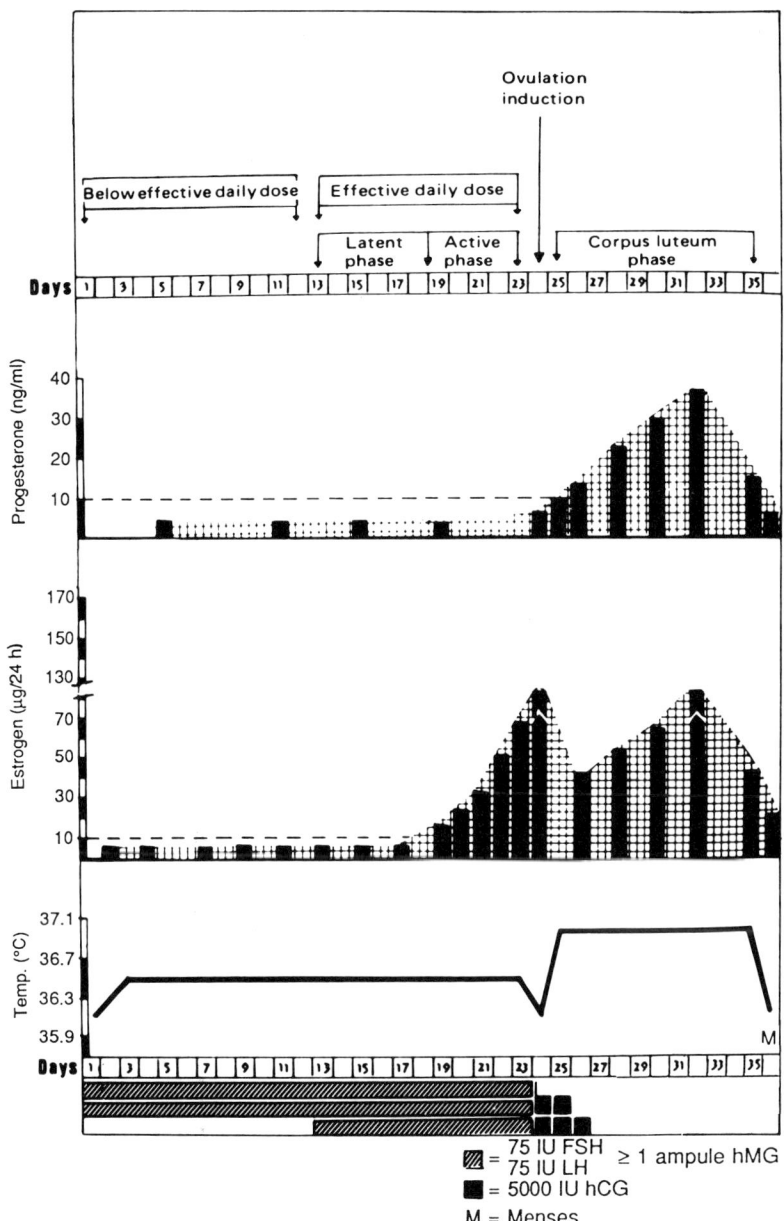

Figure 1

gesterone clearly indicate ovarian hyperactivity. Estrogen and progesterone concentrations exceed physiological levels 2–3-fold. It is obviously impossible to mimic physiological conditions by one or two injections of hMG per day. The FSH/LH ratio in commerically available hMG preparations is of the

97

Table 1 Fetal outcome

	n	%
Pregnancies	1471	100
Singletons	851	58
Twins	179	12
Triplets	105	7
Abortions	336	23

order of 1:1. It is still a matter of debate whether modifications with high FSH and low or missing LH activity are advantageous for certain conditions. Even attempts to administer hMG in a pulsatile fashion have failed to restore normal ovarian function. During three decades of clinical experience, the 1:1 FSH/LH ratio has proved to be clinically effective and there is no convincing evidence that modifications are superior in terms of pregnancy rate or ovarian hyperstimulation.

CLINICAL RESULTS

Data collected from nine different centers covering more than 3000 patients treated in almost 10000 cycles report on 1184 pregnancies, accounting for a pregnancy rate of 35%. Related to treatment cycles, however, the pregnancy rate decreases to approximately 12%.

The data in terms of pregnancy outcome, single and multiple births and abortion rate are listed in Table 1. These figures are realistic and correspond well with our own results. Since these data clearly indicate the potentials, the limits and the risks of hMG/hCG therapy, they can be helpful in counselling infertility patients.

Ovarian hyperstimulation is the main complication associated with gonadotropin therapy. This subject has been reviewed by Schenker and Weinstein[8]. The pathophysiology of this phenomenon is still unknown. Prostaglandins may be involved causing increased permeability of the capillaries. The syndrome of ovarian hyperstimulation is classified according to the severity of the clinical symptoms. Severe hyperstimulation is associated with cystic enlargement of the ovaries and an acute shift of fluid from the intravascular compartment to the peritoneal and pleural cavity, causing hypovolemia, hemoconcentration, decreased renal perfusion and intravascular clotting. These conditions can be life-threatening. Therapy should be directed to prevent the development of hypovolemia with low molecular dextran infusions and appropriate electrolyte substitution. Heparin treatment may be required. In severe cases, even peritoneal and pleural drainage may be necessary. Abdominal surgery should be avoided and is only justified in very rare instances.

REFERENCES

1. Gemzell, C. (1965). Induction of ovulation with human gonadotropins. *Rec. Prog. Horm. Res.*, **21**, 179

2. Bettendorf, G., Apostolakis, M. and Voigt, K.D. (1962). Darstellung von Gonadotropin aus menschlichen Hypophysen und klinisch experimentellen Studien mit menschlichem hypophysären Gonadotropinen. *Acta Endocrinol.*, **41**, 13
3. Crooke, A.C., Butt, W.R., Palmer, R.F., Morris, R., Logan, R. and Annon, C.A. (1963). Clinical trial of human gonadotropins. *J. Obstet. Gynaecol. Br. Cwlth.*, **163**, 604
4. Lunenfeld, B. (1963). Treatment of anovulation by human gonadotropins. *Int. J. Gynecol. Obstet.*, **1**, 153
5. Schwartz, M. and Jewelewicz, R. (1981). The use of gonadotropins for induction of ovulation. *Fertil. Steril.*, **35**, 3
6. Breckwoldt, M., Geisthövel, F., Neulen, J. and Schillinger, H. (1988). *Fertil. Steril.*, **49**, 713
7. Insler, V., Melmed, H., Eichenbrenner, I., Serr, D.M. and Lunenfeld, B. (1972). The cervical score – a simple semiquantitative method for monitoring of the menstrual cycle. *Int. J. Gynecol. Obstet.*, **10**, 223
8. Schenker, J.G. and Weinstein, D. (1979). Ovarian hyperstimulation syndrome: a current survey. In Wallach, E.E. and Kempers, R.D. (eds.) *Modern Trends in Infertility and Conception Control*, p. 177. (Baltimore: Williams and Wilkins)

11

Pulsatile GnRH treatment for induction of ovulation in polycystic ovary syndrome

J. Schoemaker, C.W. Burger and M.M. van Weissenbruch

On the basis of the findings of Knobil and colleagues, extensively reviewed in the 1980 volume of *Recent Progress in Hormone Research*[1], Leyendecker[2], in 1978, started a new therapy for induction of ovulation in women with hypothalamic amenorrhea, by means of pulsatile administration of the hypothalamic peptide gonadotropin releasing hormone (GnRH). This therapy is based on the fact that continuous administration of GnRH, s.c. or i.v., causes desensitization of the pituitary. Only when GnRH is administered in small doses every 60–120 min can a sustained, albeit intermittent, release of LH and FSH be achieved.

Pulsatile administration of GnRH is accomplished by portable computer-ized infusion pumps, of which a number of different types are now available on the market. GnRH may be administered subcutaneously as well as intra-venously, the latter giving slightly better results. The GnRH dose may vary between 2 and 20 μg per pulse. Continued pulsatile administration of GnRH leads to induction of ovulation in most women with a hypogonadotropic amenorrhea of suprapituitary origin. The ovulation rate is as high as 95–98% and 80% of the women have achieved pregnancy after 5 months of treatment. For an extensive update of these data the reader is referred to ref. 3.

The success of GnRH therapy in patients with hypothalamic amenorrhea gave investigators hope that the treatment of other endocrinological disorders with pulsatile GnRH therapy might be successful as well. These disorders included the luteal phase defect, abnormal cervical mucus, delayed puberty, hyperprolactinemic amenorrhea and clomiphene citrate (CC)-resistant poly-cystic ovary syndrome (PCOS). The complications of human menopausal gonadotropin/human chorionic gonadotropin (hMG/hCG) therapy, especially in the latter, initially led to the incidental use of GnRH for ovulation induction in this type of disorder. The intact negative feedback of steroids during GnRH therapy, in contrast to hMG/hCG therapy, should result in minimal side-effects in women with CC-resistant PCOS. Hammond

Note: Parts of this chapter have been previously published[23,24] and have been used with permission of the publisher[23] and the authors[23,24].

and colleagues[4] in 1979 administered GnRH with a dose of 1000 μg 3 times per day. Six patients were treated, and two out of 16 treatment units (TUs) resulted in ovulation.

Table 1 summarizes the clinical results of ovulation induction with GnRH in patients with PCOS. Although it is very tempting to compare these studies, it must be emphasized that the criteria for PCOS used by the different investigators were not uniform. Furthermore, the definition of clomiphene citrate resistance in most cases was poorly described. Therefore, these studies may include CC-resistant patients with PCOS about whom it is not known whether they had been treated with the maximum dose of 1000 mg of CC. Patients with the latter maximum dose of CC may respond less satisfactorily to GnRH. Finally, in treating infertility, other factors such as tubal patency or male infertility may, of course, play an important role. Correction for these factors has to be made if data are to be compared at all.

From 1984 on, the interest in GnRH therapy in PCOS has been regained, after the disappointing results of Hammond et al.[4] in 1979. Since the 20 μg GnRH pulse dose was sufficient in hypothalamic amenorrhea, the same pulse dose was usually applied to patients with PCOS. The 90-min pulse interval was the most favored. However, the number of patients with PCOS treated with pulsatile GnRH is too limited to draw statistically significant conclusions. Molloy et al.[13] described only one patient with PCOS treated with pulsatile GnRH. The greatest number of patients, 22, has been described by Tucker et al.[10]. The ovulation rate per number of TUs varied from 0 to 83% with a median percentage of 45. The ovulation rate per number of women treated varied from 0 to 100% with a median of 32% (Table 1). It is surprising that several investigators scored a relatively high success, with respect to ovulation as well as to pregnancy[8,10,18], whereas others found no ovulation at all[9,13,16]. This discrepancy remains unsolved but it may be caused by the fact that the patients were not selected according to the same definition of PCOS. Many authors reported multiple ovulatory TUs, without pregnancies[4,7,18,12,19,20].

Pregnancy rates, varying from 13 to 53%, have been reported by four groups of investigators[5,8,11,17], with a median of 25%. But if it is taken into account that studies without pregnancies were not included, pregnancy rates considerably decrease to a range of 0–53% with a median of 0%! So, only a few patients with PCOS treated with GnRH may respond to GnRH therapy with a pregnancy. Furthermore, patients with PCOS who are CC-resistant have a long history of infertility, indicating that in these patients other factors too may have an impact on the fertilization rate.

In order to further elucidate the effectiveness of pulsatile GnRH therapy in PCOS patients a further study was undertaken. Eleven healthy women with CC-resistant PCOS were recruited for the study and treated for 85 treatment units (either an ovulatory induced cycle or a period of treatment with a constant pulse dose and pulse interval). They were between 25 and 35 years of age and not all of them were free from other infertility factors. GnRH was administered in a pulse dose of either 5, 10, 20 or 40 μg/min, with a pulse interval of 60, 90 or 120 min.

Seventy four (87%) presumed ovulations occurred in nine (82%) patients. Three patients became pregnant. Of these, one had two spontaneous

Table 1 Clinical results of ovulation induction with pulsatile GnRH in women with PCOS

Reference	Pulse dose (μg)	Pulse interval (min)	Route of administration	Number of patients	Total no. of TUs	Ovulatory TUs	Ovulation rate (%) A	B	Luteal support	P/MP/A	PR	OHSS	Phlebitis
4	1000	480	s.c.	6	18	2	11	33	GnRH	0/0/0	0		
5	10/20	90	i.v.	15	42	29	69	66	GnRH	8/0/*	53		
6	10/20	90	i.v.	8	8	5	62.5	63	GnRH	1/0/*	13		
7	5	90	i.v.	4	—*	16	—	—**	GnRH	0	0		
8	2–20	90/180	i.v.	4	18	1	6	25	GnRH	0	0		
9	1–10	96/180	i.v.	*	5	0	0	0	hCG	0	0		
10	10–25	90	i.v.	22	18	11	65	—	GnRH/ hCG	5/0/2	—		
11	5–20	90	i.v.	16	44	26	59	69	hCG	5/–/–	35		occasional
12	0.025/kg	90	i.v.	4	6	5	83	100	—	0	0		
13	6–20	60	i.v./s.c.	1	1	0	0	0		0	0		
14	4–15	90/120	i.v.	*	18	9	50	—	hCG	3/–/–	—		
15	8–20	90/124	i.v.	*	18	5	38	56	GnRH	0	0		16 x
16	15	90	s.c.	6	8	0	0	0	hCG	0	0		
			i.v.	4	4	2	50	—	hCG	0	0		
17	5–20	120/180	i.v./s.c.	8	22	4	64	63	hCG	1	20		
18	20	90	i.v.	13	20	12	66	—	hCG	4/0/2	—	1	
19	5–20	120	i.v.	3	5	2	40	33	hCG	0	0		
20	20–40	120	s.c.	4	12	2	17	25	GnRH	0	0		

*Unknown; A, percentage of TUs becoming ovulatory; B, percentage of women becoming ovulatory; **, total number of TUs unknown, therefore ovulation rate is unknown; P/MP/A, number of pregnancies/multiple pregnancies/spontaneous abortions; PR, percentage of women becoming pregnant; OHSS, ovarian hyperstimulation syndrome grade 1 abortions before she carried her third pregnancy to term. The other two patients delivered healthy children at term also.

Treatment units lasted from 17 to 60 days. Four patients acquired relatively regular ovulatory cycles of a duration between 25 and 36 days. Two patients acquired irregular ovulatory cycles varying in length from 28 to 48 days. Three patients had too few cycles to judge regularity. The duration of the treatment unit was not influenced by the pulse dose or by the pulse interval.

The constant estrogen phase (CEP), i.e. the period of relatively constant estrogen secretion from the day of the start of therapy until the day after which estrogen excretion began to increase progressively, ranged between 0 and 94 days. This CEP was not influenced by the pulse dose or the pulse interval or by the accumulated number of TUs. The range of the CEP in ovulatory treatment units was 0–36 days. This led us to the conclusion that, if pulsatile GnRH is used for ovulation induction in PCOS, a rise in estrogens should be observed within 36 days of treatment. If not, treatment should be discontinued at that point because of the low chance of ovulation beyond that time.

The progressive estrogen increase phase (PEIP), i.e. the period from the last day of constant estrogen excretion, until and including the day of maximum estrogen excretion, varied between 3 and 11 days, with one exception of 18 days. Although they were higher in stimulated cycles, the profiles of estrogen excretion during the PEIP were similar to a control group of nine normally cycling women. Luteal phase length and total pregnanediol excretion were not different from those in normal cycles.

No hyperstimulation syndrome occurred in any of the 85 TUs performed.

From these studies we concluded that ovulation induction with pulsatile GnRH is possible with a low complication rate, although the ovulation rate is not as high as in hypothalamic amenorrhea. Treatment with pulsatile GnRH changes the incidence of ovulatory cycles in PCOS but does not really change the pathological mechanisms of the disease.

The varying length of the constant estrogen phase, that is the phase in which apparently nothing happens with respect to follicular growth, is frustrating both to the patient and to the doctor and may also be responsible for the lack of popularity of this treatment.

Recent developments in other areas of ovulation induction may have paved the way for a new approach to the problem of what initiates follicular growth. In a pharmacodynamic and pharmacokinetic study in which 'pure' follicle stimulating hormone (FSH) was compared to hMG, we studied the plasma levels which stimulated follicular growth in hypogonadotropic patients, in regularly cycling women whose gonadotrophs had been suppressed by a continuous infusion of GnRH, and in women suffering from polycystic ovary syndrome, during induction of ovulation. Gonadotropins were administered i.v. by a portable infusion pump (Autosyringe, Hooksett, N.H., model AS6H). Plasma FSH levels were determined daily as were LH levels and 24-h urinary estrogen and pregnanediol excretion. At daily sonography of the ovaries we were able to definitely recognize the same follicle day after day, once it had reached a diameter of 12 mm.

Chikazawa et al.[21] showed that at a size of 5 mm the growing follicle has already been selected as a dominant one. At this size it is thus already FSH-dependent. During the follicular phase of a cycle, follicles tend to grow with a speed of approximately 2 mm in diameter per day, both in spontaneous and stimulated cycles[22]. Using this growth speed, we retrospectively calculated the time at which the follicle has probably had a size of 5 mm. The FSH level at this moment in time obviously had been able to stimulate follicular growth. Had this time been preceded by a period in which a lower dose of FSH had been given to the same patient, the FSH level at such a time was recognized as one at which follicular growth had not been stimulated.

Evaluation of such levels showed that, in hypogonadotropic women, follicular growth was only stimulated by FSH levels greater than 7.8 U/l (Amerlex RIA, Amersham, UK, MRC 68/39). In 20 cycles there was no exception to this rule. Moreover, in 12 cycles stimulated in normally cycling women under suppression of a continuous GnRH infusion, the same absolute discriminating level was found. In this group there were no exceptions to the rule either.

Evaluating these stimulatory and non-stimulatory FSH levels in 119 cycles in women with PCOS, however, an overlap appeared to exist. The absolute stimulatory and absolute non-stimulatory levels here appeared to be discriminated by a zone ranging from 6.3 to 9.8 U/l, in which FSH levels might be stimulatory in one cycle and non-stimulatory in another. This overlap appeared to be caused by an inter- as well as an intra-individual variability in sensitivity of stimulated follicles. As the effect of FSH on the follicle may be modulated by different growth factors such as insulin, insulin-like growth factor, transforming growth factors α and β, and epidermal growth factor, we postulate that this variability in sensitivity of follicles in polycystic ovary syndrome may be caused at least in part by a variability in the secretion of such growth factors in women suffering from PCOS.

In the previously discussed 85 treatment units in induction of ovulation by pulsatile GnRH in PCOS women we measured FSH daily in 20 such cycles, 16 of those being ovulatory and four anovulatory. In applying the knowledge of threshold levels to these 20 cycles it appeared that at least three of the four anovulatory cycles had low FSH levels. Although no ultrasound monitoring of these cycles had been performed, thereby excluding the possibility of a direct comparison with the gonadotropin stimulated cycles, these findings at least suggest that the GnRH-stimulated cycles had remained anovulatory because of a failure of the FSH level to reach the threshold necessary for follicular growth.

On the basis of these findings, we hypothesize that if follicular growth can be initiated by, for example, adding FSH to the GnRH, in the beginning of treatment a more consistent ovulatory response pattern might be obtained, while at the same time the very low hyperstimulation rate, as found in pulsatile GnRH stimulation, might be preserved.

REFERENCES

1. Knobil, E. (1980). The neuroendocrine control of the menstrual cycle. In Greep, R.O. (ed.) *Recent Progress in Hormone Research*, Vol. 36, pp. 53–88. (New York, London, Toronto, Sydney, San Francisco: Academic Press)

2. Leyendecker, G. (1979). The pathophysiology of hypothalamic ovarian failure. *Eur. J. Obstet. Gynecol. Reprod. Biol.*, **9**, 175–86
3. Coelingh Bennink, H.J.T., Dogterom, A.A., Lappöhn, R.E., Rolland, R. and Schoemaker, J. (1986). Pulsatile GnRH 1985. In *Proceedings of the 3rd Ferring Symposium*, September 1985, Noordwijk. (Haarlem: Ferring Publication)
4. Hammond, C.B., Wiebe, R.H., Haney, A. and Yancy, S.G. (1979). Ovulation induction with luteinizing hormone-releasing hormone in amenorrheic, infertile women. *Am. J. Obstet. Gynecol.*, **135**, 924
5. Coelingh Bennink, H.J.T. (1984). The effect of pulsatile intravenous administration of GnRH on gonadotropin secretion in polycystic ovarian disease. *Fertil. Steril.*, **41**, 34S, Abstr. 160
6. Coelingh Bennink, H.J.T. (1984). Induction of ovulation by pulsatile intravenous administration of GnRH in polycystic ovarian disease. *Fertil. Steril.*, **41**, 34S, Abstr. 80
7. Rolland, R., Lorijn, R.H.W. and Willemsen, W.N.P. (1984). Chronic, intermittent administration of gonadotropin-releasing hormone (LHRH) in infertile women with different cycle abnormalities. *J. Steroid Biochem.*, **20**, 1402
8. Loucopoulos, A., Ferin, M., van de Wiele, R.L., Dyrenfurth, I., Linkie, D., Yeh, M. and Jewelewicz, R. (1984). Pulsatile administration of gonadotropin releasing hormone for induction of ovulation. *Am. J. Obstet. Gynecol.*, **148**, 895
9. Liu, J.H. and Yen, S.C.C. (1984). The use of gonadotropin releasing hormone for induction of ovulation. *Clin. Obstet. Gynecol.*, **27**, 975
10. Tucker, M., Adams, J. and Mason, W.P. (1984). Multiple cystic ovarian disease. Presented at *7th International Congress of Endocrinology*, Quebec City, Canada
11. Berg, D., Mickan, H., Michael, S., Döring, K., Gloning, K., Jänicke, F. and Rjosk, H.K. (1983). Ovulation and pregnancy after pulsatile administration of gonadotropin releasing hormone. *Arch. Gynaekol.*, **233**, 205
12. Ory, S.J., London, S.N., Tyrey, L.T. and Hammond, C.B. (1985). Ovulation induction with pulsatile gonadotropin-releasing hormone administration in patients with polycystic ovarian syndrome. *Fertil. Steril.*, **43**, 20
13. Molloy, B.G., Hancock, K.W. and Glass, M.R. (1985). Ovulation induction in clomiphene nonresponsive patients: the place of pulsatile gonadotropin-releasing hormone in clinical practice. *Fertil. Steril.*, **43**, 26
14. Bringer, J., Hedon, B., Jaffiol, C., Nicolau, S., Gibert, F., Cristol, P., Orsetti, A., Viala, J.L. and Mirouze, J. (1985). Influence of the frequency of gonadotropin-releasing hormone (GnRH) administration on ovulatory responses in women with anovulation. *Fertil. Steril.*, **44**, 42
15. Bringer, J., Hedon, B., Gibert, F., Mares, P., Jaffiol, C., Orsetti, A., Boutes, C., Viala, J.L. and Mirouze, J. (1986). Treatment of anovulation by HMG or GnRH: contribution of a cross-over randomized study to rational management of PCO. Pulsatile GnRH 1985. In *Proceedings of the 3rd Ferring Symposium*, September 1985, Noordwijk, p. 171. (Haarlem: Ferring Publication)
16. Ross, L.D., Robertson, G., Milton, P.J.D. and Blows, R. (1985). The induction of ovulation using pulsatile luteinizing hormone releasing hormone in clinical practice. *Br. J. Obstet. Gynaecol.*, **92**, 815
17. Phansey, S.A., Toffle, R., Curtin, J., Nagel, T.C., Tagatz, G.E., Barnes, M.A. and Nair, R. (1985). Alternative indications for pulsatile gonadotropin-releasing hormone therapy in infertile women. *Fertil. Steril.*, **44**, 589
18. Birkhäuser, M.H. and Huber, P. (1986). Pathophysiological aspects and clinical results of ovulation induction by pulsatile intravenous administration of GnRH in polycystic ovary syndrome (PCO-S). Pulsatile GnRH 1985. In *Proceedings of the 3rd Ferring Symposium*, September 1985, Noordwijk, p. 171. (Haarlem: Ferring Publication)
19. Saffan, D. and Seibel, M.M. (1986). Ovulation induction with subcutaneous pulsatile gonadotropin releasing hormone in various ovulatory disorders. *Fertil. Steril.*, **45**, 475
20. Hurwitz, A., Rosenn, B., Palti, Z., Ebstein, B., Har-Nir, R. and Ron, M. (1986). The hormonal response of patients with polycystic ovarian disease to subcutaneous low frequency pulsatile administration of luteinizing hormone releasing hormone. *Fertil. Steril.*, **46**, 378
21. Chikazawa, K., Araki, S. and Tamada, T. (1985). Morphological and endocrinological studies of follicular development during the human menstrual cycle. *J. Clin. Endocrinol. Metab.*, **62**, 305–13

22. Ritchie, W.G.M. (1985). Ultrasound in the evaluation of normal and induced ovulation. *Fertil. Steril.*, **43**, 167

23. Schoemaker, J., Burger, C.W. and Lambalk, C.B. (1987). Is GnRH infusion a treatment of polycystic ovarian disease (PCOD)? In Selam, J.L. and Ensminger, W.D. (eds.) *Infusion Systems in Medicine*, pp. 315–25. (Mount Kisco, NY, USA: Futura Publishing Company Inc.)

24. Burger, C.W. (1987). *Luteinizing Hormone-Releasing Hormone in Polycystic Ovary-like Disease*. Thesis Vrije Universiteit, Amsterdam. (Katwijk: A11-In)

12

Induction of ovulation with GnRH analogs and gonadotropins in polycystic ovary syndrome

R. Fleming

INTRODUCTION

The complex of abnormal endocrine environment and ovarian pathophysiology results in a low frequency of normal ovulation which is the major cause of infertility in patients with polycystic ovary syndrome (PCO). The elevated concentrations of plasma luteinizing hormone (LH) commonly associated with PCO may or may not have a specific role in the etiology of the condition and the resulting infertility, although it is likely to be responsible for the increased thecal activity. The infertility amongst PCO patients may be more directly related to LH activity, since, in the event of an apparently normal follicle proceeding to maturation, the elevated LH itself may have an adverse effect upon oocyte release[1] and viability[2]. This may be reflected in the observation that patients with oligomenorrhea and raised LH levels often show subnormal or deficient luteal phase progesterone (P) profiles when and if luteinization or 'ovulation' occurs spontaneously[3].

Treatment of PCO patients with conventional ovulation induction (human menopausal gonadotropin/human chorionic gonadotropin) (hMG/hCG) has shown disappointing pregnancy rates and high complication rates, usually due to excessive follicular development.

In the late follicular phase of the normal cycle, LH and follicle stimulating hormone (FSH) are suppressed to low levels, and luteinization and ovulation occur only after an LH surge induced by the high circulating estradiol (E_2) concentrations. During the induction of follicular development with exogenous gonadotropins (hMG) in women with functional pituitaries, elevated plasma levels of E_2 are usually observed due to the multiple follicles produced, and this steroid profile often induces LH surges and luteinization before individual follicles are of mature size (Figure 1). This process appears to be associated with a reduction in oocyte viability and pregnancy rates in an *in vitro* fertilization (IVF) program[4]. Although suppression of LH by the increasing E_2 concentrations was observed during hMG therapy in the PCO patient shown in Figure 1, a premature LH surge was seen when the largest

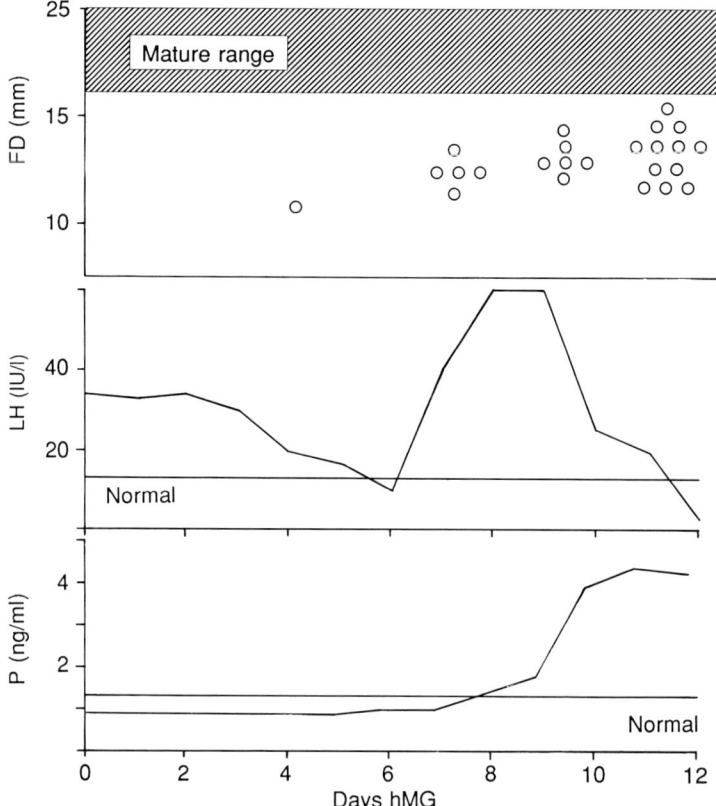

Figure 1 Profiles of progesterone (P), LH and ultrasound observations in a patient with PCO treated with hMG alone. The striped area represents the follicle diameters (FD) defining normal, mature preovulatory size. The normal maximum progesterone concentration on day 0 of the normal cycle is 1.5 ng/ml

follicle was only about 15 mm in diameter. This surge was rapidly followed by elevation of plasma progesterone concentration, and this phenomenon may be expected after the induction of multiple follicular growth in any patient with a functional pituitary.

In patients with hypogonadotropic hypogonadism, LH surges and premature luteinization do not occur, and hMG/hCG therapy is a highly successful procedure with high ovulation and pregnancy rates[5]. Therefore, is the difficulty in treating PCO patients with ovulation induction due to inappropriate LH activity during treatment cycles, or because of implicitly abnormal follicles and gametes?

Approximately 2 weeks continued treatment with gonadotropin releasing hormone analogs (GnRH-A) reversibly suppresses both bioactive and radioimmunoassayable LH, and this may therefore be used to attempt to convert the responses of PCO patients to hMG into those seen in patients with hypogonadotropic hypogonadism. This has been shown to eliminate the pre-hCG LH surge and premature luteinization, and may yield a pregnancy rate approaching that of patients with hypogonadotropic hypogonadism. It may also reduce the incidence of ovarian hyperstimulation – a complication often associated with PCO patients.

METHODS

Patients

All PCO patients showed oligomenorrhea (usual cycle length > 41 days) with elevated plasma LH concentrations (mean of more than two samples), high or high/normal androstenedione levels, normal husband semen analyses, and infertility of more than 3 years' duration. In all cases laparoscopy revealed a normal pelvis, and clomiphene citrate therapy for a minimum of 12 months had failed to achieve a pregnancy.

GnRH-A administration

The GnRH-A used was the nasal spray (buserelin; Hoechst UK Ltd.) which was both effective and convenient for the variable durations required. The original dose was $5 \times 100 \, \mu g/day$ although the manufacturer's recommended dose of $4 \times 300 \, \mu g/day$ was equally effective. Buserelin treatment was initiated at least 14 days prior to the initiation of hMG therapy. As shown in the example in Figure 2, the agonistic 'flare' effect of treatment initiation often caused some ovarian activity, and the ensuing menstrual bleed could be used as a clinical marker to indicate that the gonadotropins and follicular development were effectively suppressed, so that hMG therapy could be started.

Ovulation induction and monitoring

Daily injections of hMG were administered until follicular maturity was diagnosed at which point hCG was administered (day 0). The initial dose of hMG was 2 ampules/day, and daily plasma E_2 estimations allowed titration of the dose against responses. hCG (5000 IU) was administered when follicular maturity (follicular diameter > 17 mm) was diagnosed by ovarian ultrasonography only if the E_2 concentration was between 750 pmol/l (250 pg/ml) and 7500 pmol/l (2500 pg/ml). Further hCG (2500 IU) was administered for luteal support on days $+3$ and $+6$ (relative to day 0) unless excessive ovarian enlargement was observed.

In the event of the day 0 criteria not being achieved, usually because of excessive E_2 produced by too many follicles, hCG was withheld while the patient was maintained on GnRH-A therapy. This was not counted as a treatment cycle. After a menstrual bleed (estrogen withdrawal; MP) and disappearance of the cysts, hMG was restarted, usually at a lower dose.

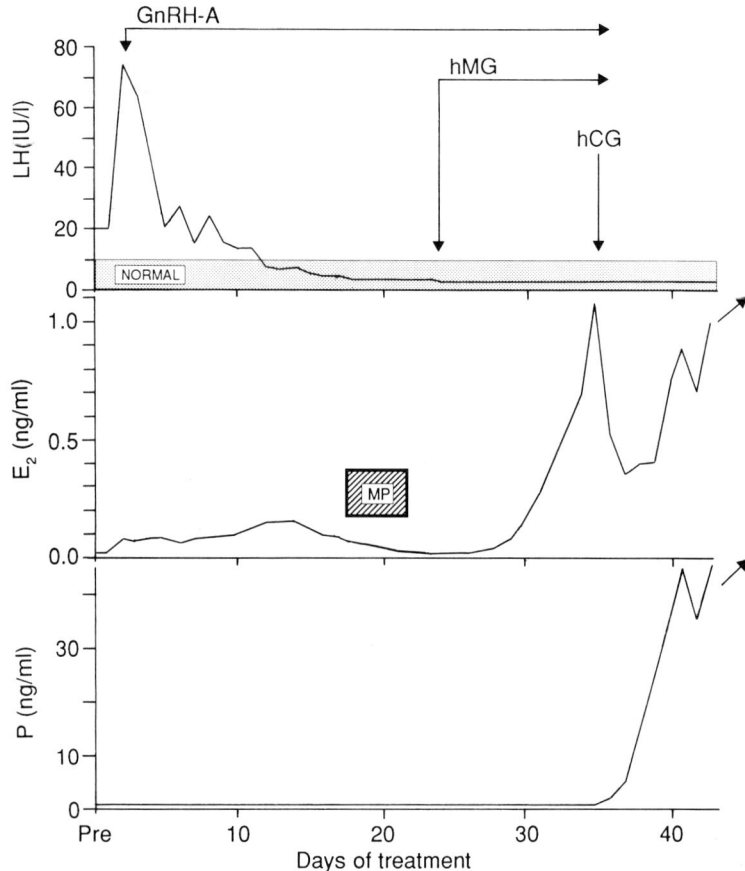

Figure 2 An example of the complete treatment procedure in one patient. The pretreatment data (Pre; mean plus SD of 2 weeks samples) is shown before the initiation of GnRH-A therapy, which is followed by hMG and hCG. Two mature sized follicles were observed when hCG was administered (day 0) and a singleton pregnancy resulted. No pre-hCG elevations in LH or progesterone (P) were observed

RESULTS

Effects of combined therapy on hormone profiles and premature luteinization

During ovulation induction in PCO patients using hMG alone, a wide variety of LH and steroid hormone profiles was observed. Premature luteinization was always seen in association with elevations of LH, and under these circumstances plasma E_2 often declined despite continued hMG treatment. Table 1 shows the results of two series of patients treated simultaneously with hMG alone or with combined therapy. The degree of stimulation was similar in both groups; E_2 on day 0 showed no difference,

Table 1 Hormone results of PCO patients treated with hMG alone or combined with GnRH-A

Therapy	n	Estradiol day 0 (pmol/l)	Premature luteinization	
			n	%
hMG alone	45	3750	15	33
Combined	20	4350	0	0

but there was a 33% incidence of premature luteinization (diagnosed when plasma progesterone rose above 1.5 ng/ml (4.5 nmol/l) before observation of a 17 mm follicular diameter) in the hMG group, and complete absence in the combined group.

Figure 3 shows the LH and progesterone profiles of 13 patients treated on both treatment schemes. They showed premature luteinization prior to hCG only in the hMG-alone cycles. The combined therapy showed suppression of both LH and progesterone until after hCG administration. These were similar profiles to those seen in ovulation induction in patients with hypogonadotropic hypogonadism.

Conception rates

The conception rates in women with PCO, randomly allocated to the two treatment schemes, during their first cycle of treatment are shown in Table 2. The group on hMG therapy showed rates consistent with other published figures, while those on combined therapy showed a significant ($p < 0.05$) improvement to 35% per treatment cycle.

Over a complete treatment course (maximum of six cycles receiving hCG), the combined therapy resulted in a pregnancy rate of 84% of patients ($n = 50$), approximately double the rates published for hMG-alone therapy in PCO by other authors[6]. Figure 4 shows that the cumulative conception profile approaches that achieved in patients with hypgonadotropic hypogonadism treated with hMG alone using the same value judgements.

The incidence of multiple pregnancy should be kept to a minimum, and so far the monitoring has been successful, since only eight (19%) of the first 42 continuing pregnancies were twins, and there was no pregnancy with more than twins.

Table 2 Comparison of the incidence of pregnancy occurring in the first cycle of treatment with either hMG alone or with combined hMG and GnRH-A therapy

Therapy	n	Pregnancies in 1st cycle	
		n	%
hMG alone	38	5	13
Combined	40	14	35*

*$p < 0.05$

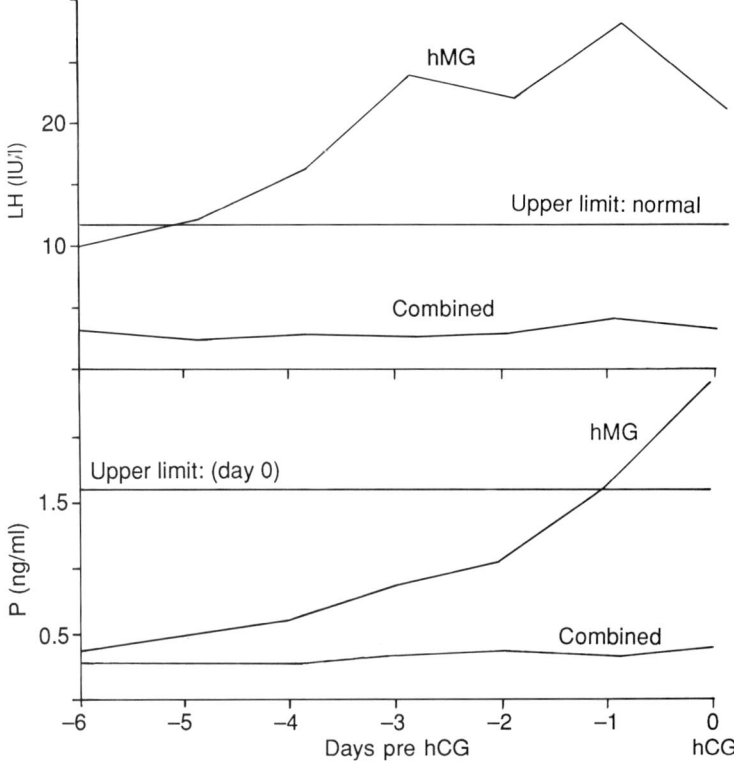

Figure 3 Profiles of mean LH and progesterone (P) during the 7 days preceding the hCG injection in 13 PCO patients who failed to conceive during the hMG therapy and who were subsequently treated with combined therapy. The combined therapy showed no pre-hCG elevations of either LH or P

OVARIAN RESPONSES TO STIMULATION

Rates of follicular growth

During the course of this work, it became apparent that patients on combined therapy responded in a similar manner to those on hMG alone. Follicles appeared to grow at similar rates and with a similar frequency of multiple follicular development.

Retrospective analyses of the distribution of large (follicular diameter > 17 mm), medium (follicular diameter 14–16.5 mm) and small (follicular diameter 10–13.5 mm) follicles present on days −5, −3 and 0 (within 20 h of hCG) were effected in the first 13 patients treated with both hMG and combined therapies. No difference was recorded either in the distribution of follicle sizes or in the rates of follicular growth over the last 6 days of hMG treatment.

Furthermore, the ratio of small follicles to large on day 0 was greater ($p < 0.05$) in the PCO patients on combined therapy and on hMG alone, than

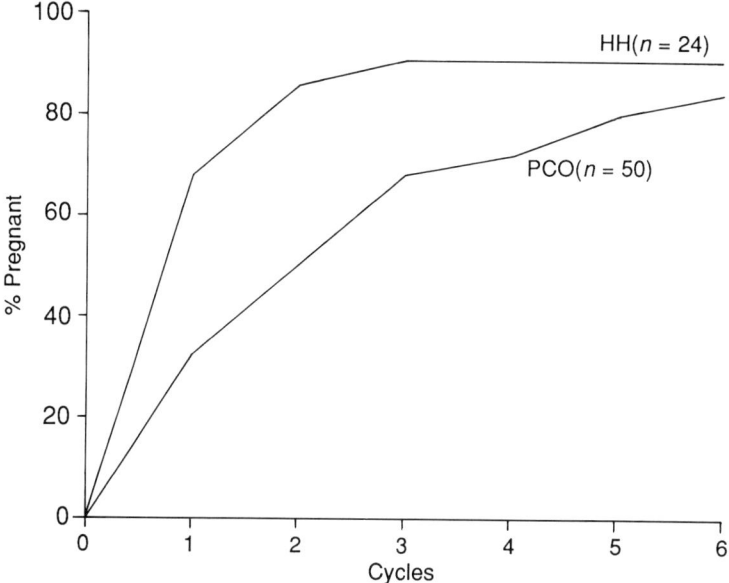

Figure 4 The cumulative conception profiles of PCO patients ($n = 50$) on combined therapy compared with that from patients with hypogonadotropic hypogonadism (HH) ($n = 24$) treated with hMG alone

in patients with hypogonadotropic hypogonadism ($n = 17$). This reflected the continued high rate of follicle recruitment in PCO patients treated with hMG compared with patients with hypogonadotropic hypogonadism.

The tendency of PCO patients to respond to hMG with excessive follicular development leads to risks of multiple ovulations and hyperstimulation and/or the withholding of the hCG injection. In a recent series of PCO patients ($n = 65$ cycles) treated with combined therapy, 12 (19%) were discontinued prior to hCG administration and the duration of GnRH-A pretreatment appears to have no influence upon this response profile.

Pregnancy loss and elevated LH

It was suggested recently[7] that increased LH concentrations during ovulation induction may be associated with an increased rate of early pregnancy loss. However, some patients in both treatment groups of PCO patients in this study suffered from early pregnancy loss, defined as failure to continue after 9 weeks' gestation (7 weeks after hCG). All were defined as clinical pregnancies, confirmed by ultrasonography between 4 and 5 weeks post-hCG.

Early pregnancy loss was confirmed in three of 19 (16%) pregnancies in the hMG-alone group (mean preovulatory LH = 11.7 IU/l) and in four out of 42 (10%) pregnancies on combined therapy (mean LH = 3.5 IU/l). There is no suggestion from these figures that suppression of LH during ovulation induction has any influence upon early pregnancy loss. As with ovarian responses, the underlying abnormality in PCO patients appears to be unrelated to the usually elevated concentrations of LH seen in this condition.

DISCUSSION

The conception rates of PCO patients treated with combined GnRH-A and hMG therapy approached that of patients with hypogonadotropic hypogonadism and eliminated complications due to LH fluctuations. This implies that the ovaries of patients with PCO contain follicles which can release normally viable oocytes given the correct gonadotropin environment.

Buserelin therapy eliminated premature luteinization and this, the most tangible consequence of LH suppression, may explain the improved pregnancy rate. There are possible theoretical benefits to be derived from reduced concentrations of LH during follicular maturation, but the evidence for this is not yet clearly delineated.

The practical clinical benefits of combined therapy are not restricted to the improved pregnancy rate, since, although the incidence of overstimulation (excessive estradiol prior to hCG) is unchanged by the LH suppression, the problems of spontaneous ovulation are avoided. Under these circumstances, hCG can be withheld and ovulation will not occur provided the GnRH-A therapy is continued. This procedure also facilitates the re-initiation of hMG therapy after a delay of approximately 2 weeks, as the follicles shrink in response to the maintained hypogonadotropism.

Evidence from follicular growth rates and the duration of hMG therapy suggest that the high rate of follicle turnover in PCO is unaffected by LH suppression, and thus the underlying metabolic disturbance is independent of LH. This means that the clinical difficulty of timing hCG administration in these patients is unaltered by GnRH-A adjuvant therapy. Thus, while the suppression of LH has no influence upon the underlying metabolic disorder of PCO, the infertility can be resolved with a high expectation of success.

REFERENCES

1. Stanger, J.D. and Yovich, J.L. (1984). Failure of human oocyte release at ovulation. *Fertil. Steril.*, **41**, 827–32
2. Stanger, J.D. and Yovich, J.L. (1985). Reduced *in vitro* fertilization of human oocytes from patients with raised basal luteinizing hormone levels during the follicular phase. *Br. J. Obstet. Gynaecol.*, **92**, 385–93
3. Sherman, B.M. and Korenman, S.G. (1974). Measurement of plasma LH, FSH, estradiol and progesterone in disorders of the menstrual cycle: the inadequate luteal phase. *J. Clin. Endocrinol. Metab.*, **39**, 145–9
4. Howles, C.M., Macnamee, M.C., Edwards, R.G., Goswamy, R. and Steptoe, P.C. (1986). Effect of high tonic levels of LH on outcome of *in vitro* fertilization. *Lancet*, **2**, 521–2
5. Lunenfeld, B. and Insler, V. (1978). The gonadotropins. In Lunenfeld, B. and Insler, V. (eds.) *Diagnosis and Treatment of Functional Infertility*, pp. 61–89. (Berlin: Gross Verlag)
6. Diamond, M.P. and Wentz, A.C. (1986). Ovulation induction with human menopausal gonadotropins. *Obstet. Gynecol. Surv.*, **41**, 480–90
7. Homburg, R., Armar, N.A., Eshel, A., Adams, J. and Jacobs, H.S. (1988). Influence of serum LH concentrations on ovulation, conception and early pregnancy loss in polycystic ovary syndrome. *Br. Med. J.*, **297**, 1024–6

13

Induction of ovulation with pulsatile GnRH in patients with polycystic ovary syndrome

M. Filicori, C. Flamigni, M.C. Meriggiola, A. Valdiserri, P. Ferrari, P. Dellai, M. Guidastri, R. Arnone and G. Cognigni

INTRODUCTION

Polycystic ovary syndrome (PCOS) is a common reproductive endocrine disorder associated with irregular menstrual cycles, anovulation, hirsutism and infertility. The endocrine pattern in these patients is often characterized by high LH, androgen and weak estrogen (estrone) levels. Obesity is often present in patients with polycystic ovary syndrome and the response to an oral glucose tolerance test may be deranged. The adrenal may contribute significantly to the excessive androgen secretion[1].

Estroprogestagens or GnRH analogs are used to suppress hypothalamic–pituitary function for the treatment of acne, hirsutism and menstrual irregularities; cyproterone acetate, an antiandrogenic progestin, is often utilized in Europe[2]. Spironolactone and corticosteroids may also be employed in specific groups of patients; a more regular ovulatory function can be obtained with these drugs[3].

Ovulation induction is used to restore fertility in anovulatory polycystic ovary syndrome patients. Clomiphene citrate appears to be relatively effective for inducing ovulation in this disorder; however, conception often may not be achieved with clomiphene citrate and more effective forms of ovulation induction may have to be used in resistant subjects. Human menopausal gonadotropins (hMG) and purified follicle stimulating hormone (FSH) are more effective than clomiphene citrate but relatively high rates of complications (ovarian hyperstimulations and multiple pregnancies) have been reported with this method[4]. Pretreatment with GnRH analogs before and during hMG administration may reduce the chance of ovarian hyperstimulation in polycystic ovary syndrome and may improve ovulation induction management.

OVULATION INDUCTION WITH PULSATILE GnRH

Spontaneous episodic gonadotropin secretion is markedly deranged in polycystic ovary syndrome[5,6]; this pattern does not appear to be capable of stimulating a physiological ovulatory function in these patients.

The administration of pulsatile gonadotropin releasing hormone (GnRH) is a highly effective ovulation induction method in hypogonadotropic hypogonadism but is often ineffective in polycystic ovary syndrome[7,8]. Most PCOS patients do not ovulate on pulsatile GnRH and the incidence of spontaneous abortion is higher[7]. Nevertheless, Coelingh Bennink[9] reported a better ovulatory rate when higher GnRH dosages were employed.

GnRH analogs can reversibly reduce gonadotropin and gonadal steroid levels, thus rendering the endocrine milieu of PCOS subjects comparable to the one of hypogonadotropic hypogonadism. We have used GnRH analogs to pretreat PCOS patients immediately before pulsatile GnRH ovulation induction to improve the endocrine and clinical response in these patients.

In our first report[10] we found that PCOS patients were characterized by an excessive gonadotropin response to pulsatile GnRH; estradiol and testosterone were also excessively elevated in the follicular phase of menstrual cycles induced in PCOS patients not pretreated with GnRH analogs. In the pulsatile GnRH cycles that were preceded by GnRH analog suppression, the pattern of reproductive hormones improved remarkably; LH was reduced both in the follicular and in the luteal phase while luteal progesterone was higher. More patients conceived in the post-analog cycles.

A more recent report from our group[11] confirmed those findings in a larger population of PCOS patients. When daily hormone levels were compared to those obtained in hypogonadotropic hypogonadism during pulsatile GnRH ovulation induction, we found the two patterns almost superimposable. This finding suggests that in PCOS also it is possible to restore physiological gonadotropin and gonadal steroid levels and to induce ovulation in most pulsatile GnRH cycles. The ovulatory and pregnancy rates of PCOS patients improved in post-analog cycles and were comparable to the rates achieved in hypogonadotropic hypogonadism. Unfortunately, we also found that the continuation of pulsatile GnRH for a second consecutive ovulation induction cycle yielded worse ovulatory results (Figure 1). Furthermore, the abortion rate was high in PCOS patients, both in pre- and post-analog cycles, suggesting that excessive gonadotropin secretion is not the major pathogenetic component of this complication.

In conclusion, pulsatile GnRH appears to be an excellent ovulation induction method both in hypogonadotropic and in PCOS patients, provided that GnRH analog suppression precedes pulsatile GnRH in PCOS. The extension of the application of this effective ovulation induction method to most anovulatory disorders should help to reduce the incidence of complications such as multiple pregnancy and ovarian hyperstimulation.

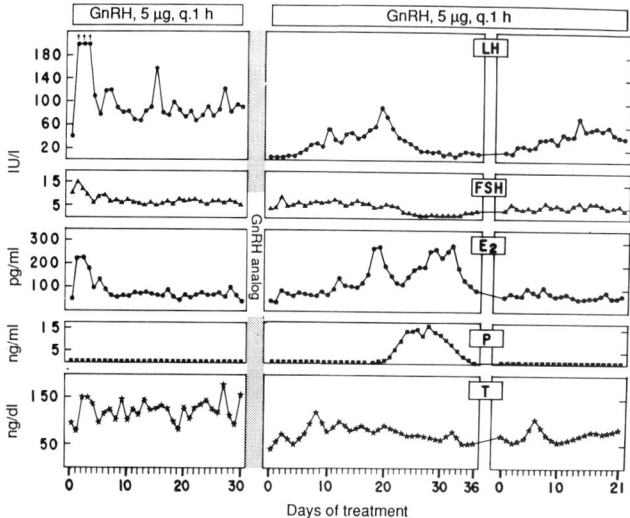

Figure 1 Daily gonadotropin and steroid concentrations in a PCOS patient treated for three cycles with pulsatile GnRH for ovulation induction. The first cycle (left panels) occurred without GnRH analog suppression; the second cycle (middle panels) was executed immediately after GnRH analog suppression, while the third cycle (right panels) occurred consecutively after the second cycle, without interrupting pulsatile GnRH administration and without repeating GnRH analog suppression. Notice that only the second cycle was ovulatory. From Filicori *et al.* (1989). *J. Clin. Endocrinol. Metab.*, 69, 825–31

ACKNOWLEDGEMENTS

We wish to thank Ms Silvia Arsento for excellent secretarial assistance.

REFERENCES

1. Loughlin, T., Cunningham, S., Moore, A., Culliton, M., Smyth, P.P.A. and McKenna, T.J. (1986). Adrenal abnormalities in polycystic ovary syndrome. *J. Clin. Endocrinol. Metab.*, **62**, 142–7
2. Hammerstein, J., Meckies, J., Leo-Rossberg, I., Moltz, L. and Zielske, F. (1975). Use of cyproterone acetate (CPA) in the treatment of acne, hirsutism and virilism. *J. Steroid Biochem.*, **6**, 827–36
3. Cumming, D.C., Yang, J.C., Rebar, R.W. and Yen, S.S.C. (1982). Treatment of hirsutism with spironolactone. *J. Am. Med. Assoc.*, **247**, 1295–8
4. Wang, C.F. and Gemzell, C. (1980). The use of human gonadotropins for the induction of ovulation in women with polycystic ovarian disease. *Fertil. Steril.*, **33**, 479–86
5. Waldstreicher, J., Santoro, N., Hall, J.E., Filicori, M. and Crowley, W.F. Jr. (1988). Hyperfunction of the hypothalamic–pituitary axis in women with polycystic ovarian disease: indirect evidence for partial gonadotroph desensitization. *J. Clin. Endocrinol. Metab.*, **66**, 165–72
6. Kazer, R.R., Kessel, B. and Yen, S.S.C. (1987). Circulating luteinizing hormone pulse frequency in women with polycystic ovary syndrome. *J. Clin. Endocrinol. Metab.*, **65**, 233–6
7. Eshel, A., Abdulwahid, N.A., Armar, N.A., Adams, J.M. and Jacobs, H.S. (1988). Pulsatile luteinizing hormone-releasing hormone therapy in women with polycystic ovary syndrome. *Fertil. Steril.*, **49**, 956–60

8. Wilson, J.M., Traub, A.I., Sheridan, B., Thompson, W. and Atkinson, A.B. (1988). Conventional dose intravenous pulsatile GnRH therapy does not induce ovulation in polycystic ovarian disease. *Acta Endocrinol. Copenh.*, **117**, 289–93

9. Coelingh Bennink, H.J.T. (1983). Induction of ovulation by pulsatile intravenous administration of LHRH in polycystic ovarian disease. In *Proceedings of the 65th Annual Meeting of the Endocrine Society* (Abstract 1)

10. Filicori, M., Campaniello, E., Michelacci, L., Pareschi, A., Ferrari, P., Bolelli, G. and Flamigni, C. (1988). Gonadotropin-releasing hormone (GnRH) analog suppression renders polycystic ovarian disease patients more susceptible to ovulation induction with pulsatile GnRH. *J. Clin. Endocrinol. Metab.*, **66**, 327–33

11. Filicori, M., Flamigni, C., Campaniello, E., Valdiserri, A., Ferrari, P., Meriggiola, M.C., Michelacci, L. and Pareschi, A. (1989). The abnormal response of polycystic ovarian disease patients to exogenous pulsatile gonadotropin-releasing hormone: characterization and management. *J. Clin. Endocrinol. Metab.*, **69**, 825–31

14

New concepts in GnRH-associated superovulation for polycystic ovary syndrome in assisted reproduction programs

R.W. Shaw and N. Amso

INTRODUCTION

It is perhaps not surprising, given the problems experienced in subjects with polycystic ovary syndrome (PCO) in attempts to stimulate follicular growth for ovulation induction, that these problems should be further amplified in attempting superovulation for assisted reproduction. The aims of superovulation regimes are (1) to maximize the number of follicles which mature, (2) to minimize the degree of asynchrony amongst developing follicles, and (3) to minimize the deleterious effects of the abnormal follicular environment on luteal function and endometrial receptivity. The discussion which follows is an approach we have adopted with PCO patients, defined as those with oligomenorrhea, increased luteinizing hormone/follicle stimulating hormone (LH/FSH) ratios, increased androgen secretion, and classical ultrasound appearances of their ovaries.

Because of the problems that PCO patients exhibit, it is essential that they have an appropriate indication for assisted reproduction, i.e. they have, in addition to their ovulation disorder, tubal disease or male factor problems amenable to successful assisted reproduction treatment. A mere failure of previous ovulation induction regimes to achieve pregnancy is considered only as the last resort for *in vitro* fertilization (IVF).

SPECIFIC PROBLEMS WITH PCO SYNDROME

High tonic LH secretion

Many patients with PCO have high tonic LH secretion. Elevated levels of LH during the later stages of follicular growth and oocyte maturation appear to be deleterious, as suggested from *in vitro* fertilization in such patients where a reduced percentage of fertilization and reduced proportion of normally developing embryos have been reported[1,2], as well as increased early pregnancy loss[3].

Premature luteinization

The use of moderate to high doses of exogenous gonadotropin in superovulation regimes will increase the already known likelihood of a high incidence of premature luteinization observed in patients undergoing ovulation induction in PCO[4]. This has already been discussed in a previous chapter. We have found that up to 30% of treatment cycles for IVF in polycystic patients are cancelled for this reason.

Ovarian hyperstimulation syndrome (OHSS)

Ovarian hyperstimulation has an increased incidence in PCO patients undergoing stimulation with exogenous gonadotropins. The possible severity of this condition and the likelihood of recurrence in subsequent treatment cycles make these patients difficult to treat appropriately and with safety.

Poor oocyte quality

It has been suggested that the oocytes recovered following superovulation in PCO patients are of reduced quality with resultant poor embryo quality[5]. This has led to arguments in favor of replacing greater numbers of pre-embryos in patients with PCO to achieve similar pregnancy rates as non-PCO patients[6]. While poor oocyte quality can occur in cycles with moderate OHSS, our own data, utilizing frozen embryos obtained from such cycles, achieve pregnancy rates which have been comparable to those obtained in non-PCO patients undergoing frozen embryo replacement. These data reflect the problems currently experienced in trying to evaluate oocyte quality, as oocyte grading is subjective and does not indicate subsequent pre-embryo potential. Oocyte quality also depends upon the maintenance of gonadotropin stimulation and exposure to appropriate levels of LH and FSH. Poor fertilization rates may well reflect poor laboratory conditions rather than specific problems with the oocytes in PCO patients.

STIMULATION PROTOCOLS FOR IVF IN PCO PATIENTS

A number of different stimulation protocols appropriate to PCO patients have been utilized in assisted reproduction programs. However, there is a high incidence of cancellation in the group overall because of premature luteinization and it would seem appropriate to adopt in the first instance protocols that are likely to control endogenous gonadotropin secretion by utilizing combination treatments of pituitary desensitization with the use of GnRH agonists. The rationale for down-regulation in assisted reproduction programs is that this may achieve recruitment of more mature follicles, while allowing suppression of a single dominant follicle, and the abolition of any endogenous LH surge and premature luteinization. In addition, they offer logistic and organizational advantages with regard to oocyte recovery timing. As outlined later in this chapter, similar protocols may offer other specific advantages for PCO patients. Several questions still remain to be answered in the use of such protocols: (1) whether treatment initiation in the luteal or early follicular phase is more advantageous; (2) particularly in PCO patients, the duration of the suppression and the criteria for achieving adequate suppression; and (3) the timing of commencement of exogenous gonadotropins. In addition, an inadequate luteal phase is likely to develop unless appropriate luteal phase support is utilized. It would seem sensible, since OHSS is likely to develop to a more severe degree with exposure to hCG, that luteal phase support in PCO patients for assisted reproduction would best be achieved by giving progestogens rather than supplemental doses of hCG.

PROBLEMS ARISING WITH GnRH CYCLES

Cyst formation

A significant proportion of patients undergoing assisted reproduction following down-regulation develop follicular or luteal cysts during the initial agonistic phase of analog administration prior to down-regulation being appropriately achieved. This is found in approximately 8–10% of treatment cycles. A baseline scan is therefore necessary prior to commencement of gonadotropin treatment, followed by aspiration of the cysts under ultrasound control if they are present.

Problems with follicular growth patterns

It is always wise to commence treatment with low-dose gonadotropins in these patients to establish individual patient sensitivity and response. However, some individuals treated initially with 1 and even 2 ampules of hMG demonstrate no follicular growth or a failure to maintain or sustain growth of follicles after 7–10 days' stimulation, perhaps indicating that the threshold for initiation and maintenance of follicular growth has not been exceeded in these patients. An adequate response should be elicited within 7–10 days of commencing exogenous gonadotropin treatment. This is demonstrated by visualizing appropriate follicular growth patterns on ultrasound scanning and from endocrine monitoring. If they have not occurred, increasing the dose of gonadotropins in that cycle may be effective or, alternatively, gonadotropins should be stopped and the cycle recommenced with a higher dosage after an induced menses. In other cycles gonadotropins may initiate growth but then fail to maintain or sustain follicular growth patterns. This may result if gonadotropin support is ceased or reduced prematurely. Thus, gonadotropins should be given daily until the time of hCG administration (see Figures 1 and 2), with no period of coasting.

In other patients, despite careful low-dose administration and monitoring, excessive follicular growth patterns may be observed, predisposing to OHSS (Figure 3). Ovarian hyperstimulation syndrome is a potentially life-threatening condition and should be avoided at all costs. Its incidence in IVF/gamete intrafallopian transfer (GIFT) stimulated cycles varies between 0.3 and 6% and develops following hCG administration. Its etiology is poorly understood. Grossly elevated levels of progesterone in the presence of hCG in the circulation appear to be an important factor in its pathogenesis. Risk factors in the development of OHSS include (1) younger age, (2) women with polycystic ovarian disease, and (3) previous history of ovarian hyperstimulation syndrome. If its development seems likely and is diagnosed just before or immediately following egg collection, then the sensible treatment is to abandon the cycle and not replace the embryos or gametes during that cycle. Treatment can then be directed towards the symptoms of the ovarian hyperstimulation syndrome more easily in the absence of possible conception.

Alternative management of OHSS

An alternative approach is to try to predict, before hCG administration or following hCG prior to embryo transfer or GIFT, those patients who are at risk of developing ovarian hyperstimulation syndrome. The development of OHSS has been observed when multifollicular growth patterns during the stimulation phase of the cycle are observed, particularly when there are more than ten viable follicles per ovary from evaluation of ovarian size with an ovarian diameter > 10 cm; and circulating estradiol levels in excess of 10 000 pmol/l. In the majority of these cases, the cycle would be abandoned and the patient continued on GnRH analog therapy throughout the putative luteal phase until menstruation occurs, hCG not being administered. Continuation of analog therapy leads to a degree of luteolysis. Such patients may experience pain from enlargement of their ovaries, but rarely experience any serious problems when hCG has not been administered, such as significant ascites, increase in platelets or hemoconcentration. When the likelihood of OHSS seems probable but not overt, an alternative approach has been adopted whereby continued monitoring occurs until appropriate maturation of leading follicles is achieved, and hCG at a moderate dose of 5000 IU has been administered, followed by collection of oocytes. The oocytes are then fertilized and the developing pre-embryos cryopreserved. The GnRH analog is then continued throughout the luteal phase and no luteal phase support is given.

Adopting this technique may result in retrieving a significant number of good quality oocytes from patients whose cycles would otherwise have been cancelled. The resulting frozen pre-embryos have been replaced during subsequent cycles with a high success rate in achieving pregnancy (see Table 1). Refinements would be to try to induce active luteolysis with agents such as anti-progesterones, and prostaglandin synthetase inhibitors may help to prevent the development of the peripheral vascular effects of OHSS.

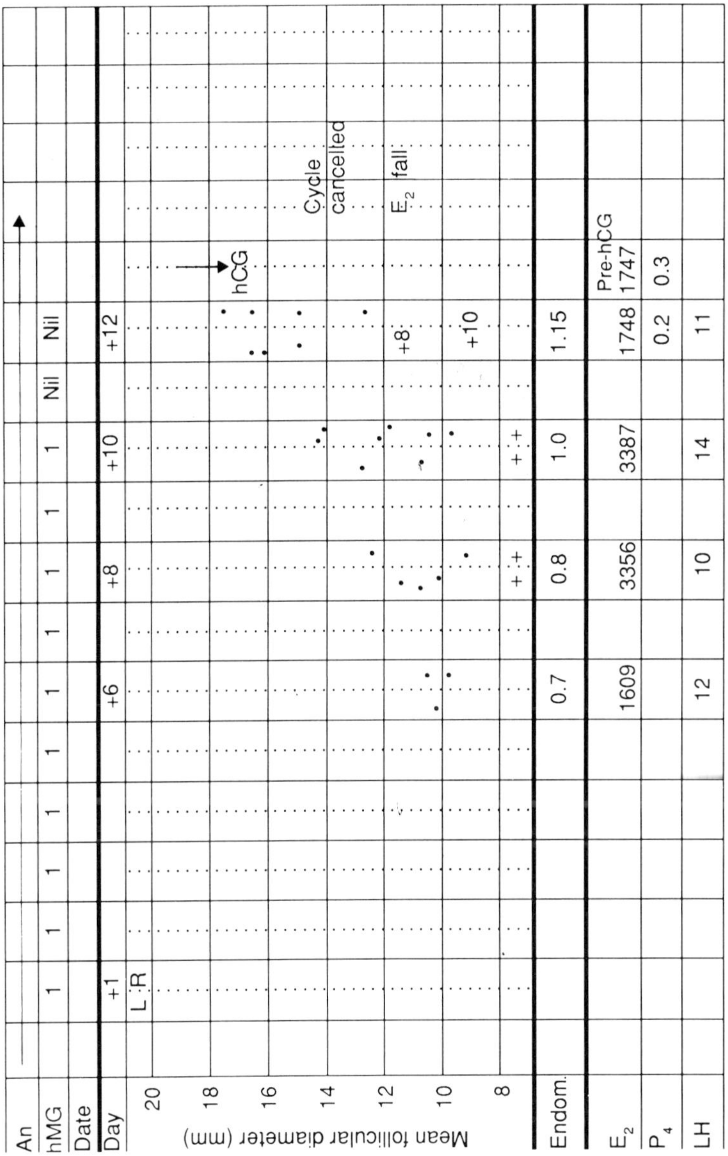

	An	hMG	Date	Day	Mean follicular diameter (mm)		Endom.	E_2	P_4	LH
	1	1	+1 L:R	+1						
	1	1								
	1	1								
	1	1								
	1	1								
	1	1	+6	+6			0.7	1609		12
	1	1	+8	+8		$+8$	0.8	3356		10
	1	1	+10	+10		$+10$	1.0	3387		14
	Nil	Nil	+12	+12	hCG	$+8$	1.15	1748 Pre-hCG 1747	0.2 0.3	11

Cycle cancelled

E_2 fall

Figure 1 Early withdrawal of exogenous gonadotropin support during combined GnRH analog (An) and Pergonal administration (hMG) resulting in slowing of follicular growth patterns and fall in serum estradiol-17β. Cycle cancelled

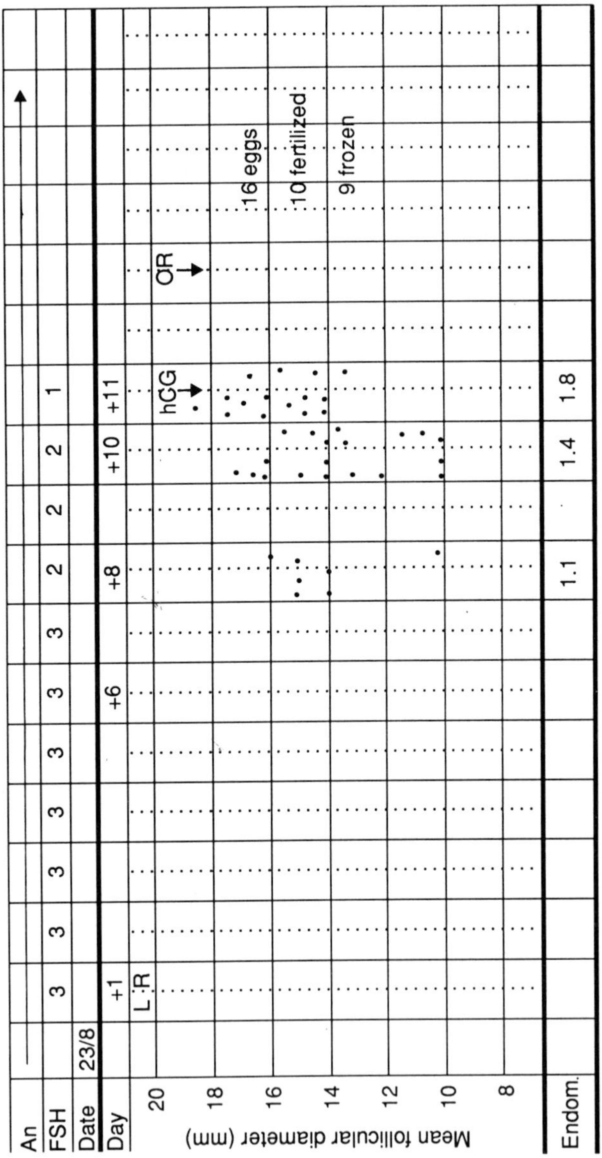

Figure 2 Close monitoring of gonadotropin dosage with reduction when leading follicle 15 mm, producing good final response. In view of multiple follicles all pre-embryos cryopreserved and no transfer performed

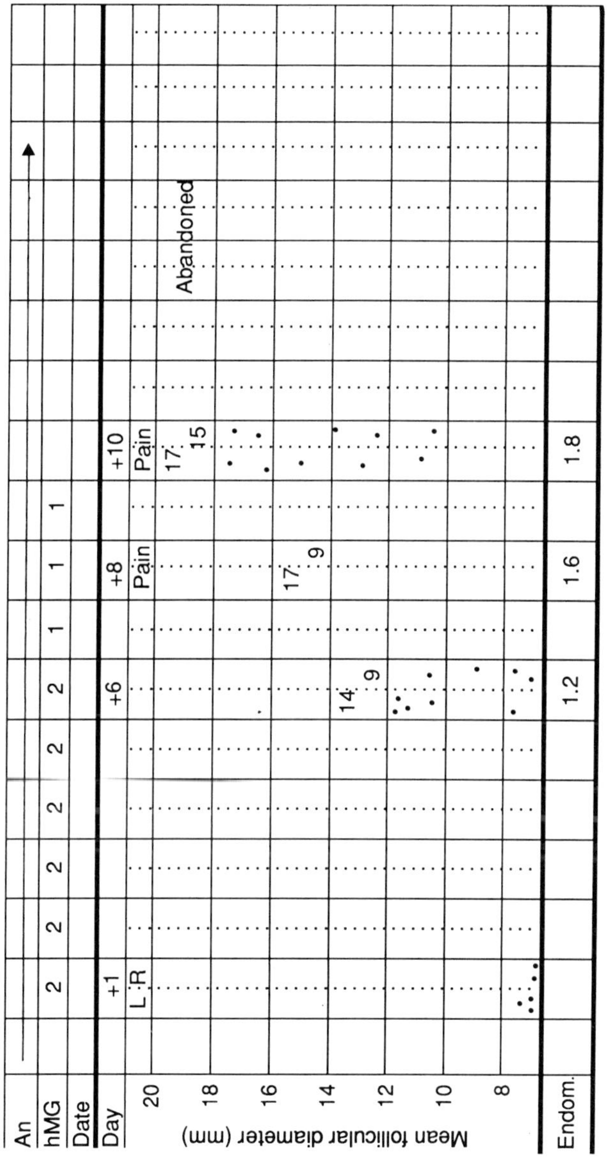

An											
hMG	2	2	2	2	2	2	2	1	1	1	1
Date											
Day	+1						+6		+8		+10	

L:R   Pain   Pain   Pain   Abandoned

Mean follicular diameter (mm): 20, 18, 16, 14, 12, 10, 8

14:9   17:9   17:15

| Endom. | | | | | | | 1.2 | | 1.6 | | 1.8 | |

Figure 3 Risk of severe OHSS developing with ovarian enlargement, discomfort and numerous large preovulatory follicles despite low-dose gonadotropins. Cycle abandoned

Table 1 Outcome of policy of elective cryopreservation of all pre-embryos in PCO patients at risk of severe OHSS

Age (years)	Number of years infertile	Viable oocytes recovered	Oocytes fertilized	Pre-embryos cryopreserved	Outcome
31	10	44	23 (52.5%)	19	Pregnant 1st FET*
34	9	37	29 (78%)	26	Pregnant 1st FET
27	3	21	12 (57%)	11	Pregnant spontaneously
29	6.5	16	12 (75%)	11	Pregnant 2nd FET

*FET = frozen embryo transfer

GUIDELINES FOR THE USE OF GONADOTROPINS IN PCO PATIENTS FOR ASSISTED REPRODUCTION

(1) Select the optimal dose of gonadotropin that maintains follicular growth at an average pace until maturity. Adjust dose downwards once the follicles grow beyond 18 mm in diameter.

(2) Combined use of GnRH analogs and gonadotropins offers many advantages and in PCO patients is probably mandatory.

(3) The development of symptoms and the signs of OHSS is dependent upon the total dosage of gonadotropins given and total duration of treatment. Discomfort and pain depend upon the size of the ovary and abandonment of treatment cycles should be considered if the clinical picture associated with ultrasound shows evidence of ovarian enlargement to > 10 cm diameter.

(4) hCG makes OHSS worse, therefore limit the ovulation dose to 5000 IU and do not administer supplementary hCG during the luteal phase but utilize progesterone to provide luteal phase support.

(5) OHSS deteriorates in pregnancy, therefore if in doubt on the day of operation for GIFT, embryo transfer or zygote intrafallopian transfer, then do not perform the transfer but freeze all pre-embryos and continue GnRH analog until menstruation occurs.

(6) Large cystic ovaries lead to complications such as hemorrhage and torsion, and therefore a close follow-up of the patient during the luteal phase is essential.

(7) OHSS is potentially fatal and due attention in the follow-up of patients should help to avoid this condition in the majority of instances.

REFERENCES

1. Stanger, J.D. and Yovich, J.L. (1985). Reduced *in-vitro* fertilization of human oocytes from patients with raised basal luteinising hormone levels during the follicular phase. *Br. J. Obstet. Gynaecol.*, **92**, 385–93

2. Howels, C.M., MacNamee, M.C., Edwards, R.G., Goswamy, R. and Steptoe, P.C. (1986). Effect of high tonic levels of luteinising hormone on outcome of *in-vitro* fertilisation. *Lancet*, **2**, 521–2

3. Homburg, R., Armar, N., Eshel, A. *et al.* (1988). Influence of serum luteinising hormone concentrations on ovulation, conception and early pregnancy loss in polycystic ovary syndrome. *Br. Med. J.*, **297**, 1024–6

4. Coutts, J.R.T. (1989). The use of LHRH analogues in ovulation induction and induction of multiple follicular growth for *in-vitro* fertilisation. In Shaw, R.W. and Marshall, J.C. (eds.) *LHRH and its Analogues*, pp. 198–213. (London, UK: Wright Publishing)

5. Pellicer, A., Ruiz, A., Castellvi, R.M., Calatayud, C., Ruis, M., Tarin, J.J., Miro, F. and Bonilla-Musoles, F. (1989). Is retrieval of high numbers of oocytes desirable in patients treated with gonadotropin-releasing hormone analogues (GnRH-a) and gonadotropins? *Hum. Reprod.*, **4**, 536–40

6. Craft, I., Al-Shawaf, T., Lewis, P., Serhal, P., Simons, E., Al-Moye, M., Fiamanya, W., Robertson, D., Shrevastav, P. and Brinsden, P. (1989). Analysis of 1071 GIFT procedures – the case for a flexible approach to treatment. *Lancet*, **1**, 1094–7

15

Beneficial effects of ovarian suppression for women with chronic hyperandrogenic anovulation

M.J. Heineman

INTRODUCTION

There is no general agreement concerning the exact definition of the polycystic ovary (PCO) syndrome. The great clinical and biochemical variability forms a major problem in appropriately defining this disease. However, without any doubt the basic symptom of the syndrome is chronic anovulation. The clinical picture is characterized by signs of androgen excess and increased anabolism.

Much interest in this disorder developed after 1935 when Stein and Leventhal[1] described a syndrome associated with polycystic ovaries. The delineation of the syndrome and the excellent results which occurred after wedge resection led to many speculations on the pathophysiology and the pathogenesis of this disease. In the original publication of Stein and Leventhal it was stated that mechanical crowding of the cortex by cysts interfered with the progress of the normal Graafian follicles to the surface of the ovary. This mechanical factor accounted for symptoms of amenorrhea and sterility. Nowadays, an endocrine disturbance is thought to be responsible for the development of this condition. The sequence of events in the maintenance of chronic hyperandrogenic anovulation in the PCO syndrome was very well described by Yen in 1976[2].

The therapeutic management of the PCO syndrome has been discussed extensively. If pregnancy is not the goal, the therapeutic approach should be suppression of the hypothalamic–pituitary–ovarian axis by the use of an estrogen–progestogen combination preparation. If the therapy is directed towards the establishment of ovulatory cycles and consequently improvement of fertility, ovulation induction by means of several preparations is possible. Clomiphene, clomiphene in combination with corticosteroids, and human menopausal gonadotropin/human chorionic gonadotropin (hMG/hCG) are often prescribed for this purpose. PCO patients have a relative shortage of follicle stimulating hormone (FSH); therefore induction of ovulation in these women may also be directed towards supplementation of this lack of FSH.

Wedge resections are nowadays not so often performed as in former days, since the occurrence of postoperative adhesions has prompted many clinicians to abandon this procedure. It has been postulated that appropriate exogenous pulsatile luteinizing hormone releasing hormone (LHRH) administration will overrule the existing inappropriate endogenous LHRH secretion which is present in PCO patients[3]. Pulsatile LHRH treatment in chronic hyperandrogenic patients has not been shown to be very successful, however. Recently, hMG/hCG therapy after down-regulation of the pituitary has been reported to be an effective approach in the treatment of clomiphene-resistant oligomenorrhea. Promising high cumulative pregnancy rates in PCO patients treated with LHRH analog/hMG/hCG have been published[4,5].

Although suppression of ovarian steroidogenesis by means of an oral contraceptive does not correct the underlying pathophysiology of the PCO syndrome, this approach may benefit patients who wish to become pregnant. The expected effects of a combination preparation for patients with the PCO syndrome are:

(1) The excessive LH production becomes normalized;

(2) Over-stimulation of the ovaries ceases;

(3) There will be a decrease of androgen production;

(4) There will be an increase of the sex hormone binding globulin level; and finally

(5) An appropriate stimulus of the endometrium and cyclic shedding, thus serving as a prophylaxis against endometrial hyperplasia, is realized.

Further progression of the disorder is not possible during the use of an estrogen–progestogen combination preparation. After withdrawal of the suppressive medication, one may expect the hormonal milieu to be more adequate for the initiation of follicular maturation.

We decided to study some endocrine aspects of ovarian suppression and follicular maturation following ovarian suppression in women with clinical features of the PCO syndrome.

MATERIALS AND METHODS

The clinical and endocrine characteristics of the PCO patients ($n = 21$) have been published previously[6]. In this group of women the LH/FSH ratio was elevated and the serum concentrations of testosterone, androstenedione, estrone and estradiol were elevated as well (Figures 1–3). Twenty of these women used the combination preparation Diane® (2 mg cyproterone acetate and 0.05 mg ethinylestradiol) for a period of 3 months in a discontinuous way.

Blood samples were collected according to a strict time schedule. The first sample was taken on the morning of the day prior to the initiation of therapy. The remaining samples were obtained after 4, 7, 11 and 14 days. After this initial period another five samples were obtained at 2-week intervals.

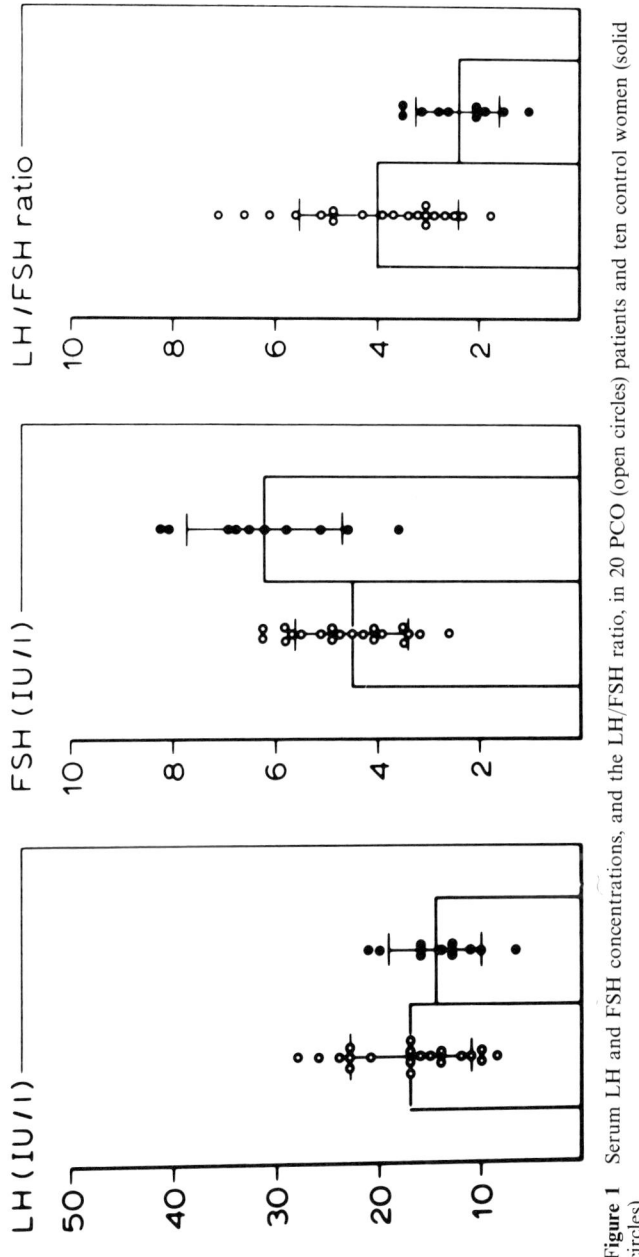

Figure 1 Serum LH and FSH concentrations, and the LH/FSH ratio, in 20 PCO (open circles) patients and ten control women (solid circles)

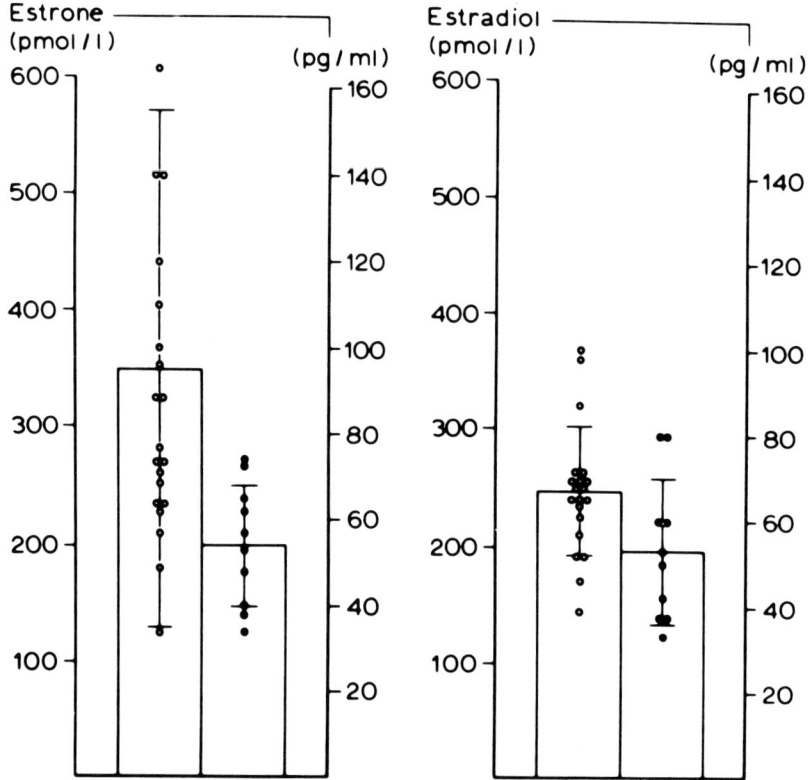

Figure 2 Serum estrone and estradiol concentrations in 20 PCO (open circles) patients and ten control women (solid circles)

Some hormonal changes related to the process of spontaneous follicular maturation and ovulation were evaluated in those PCO patients ($n = 17$) who wished to become pregnant after withdrawal of the combination preparation Diane®.

The Wilcoxon one-sample test was used to determine the effect of Diane® administration on the serum levels of the measured steroids in the PCO patients. Two-sided p values are given for all parameters.

RESULTS

During the use of the combination preparation, a gradual decrease of LH could be demonstrated. FSH levels decreased during the medication periods; however, a rapid recovery of FSH was seen after withdrawal of medication. As a consequence of these changes, the LH/FSH ratio was significantly lower at the end of the treatment period ($p = 0.008$) (Figure 4) (Table 1). The serum estrone concentration decreased during the treatment period. The estrone

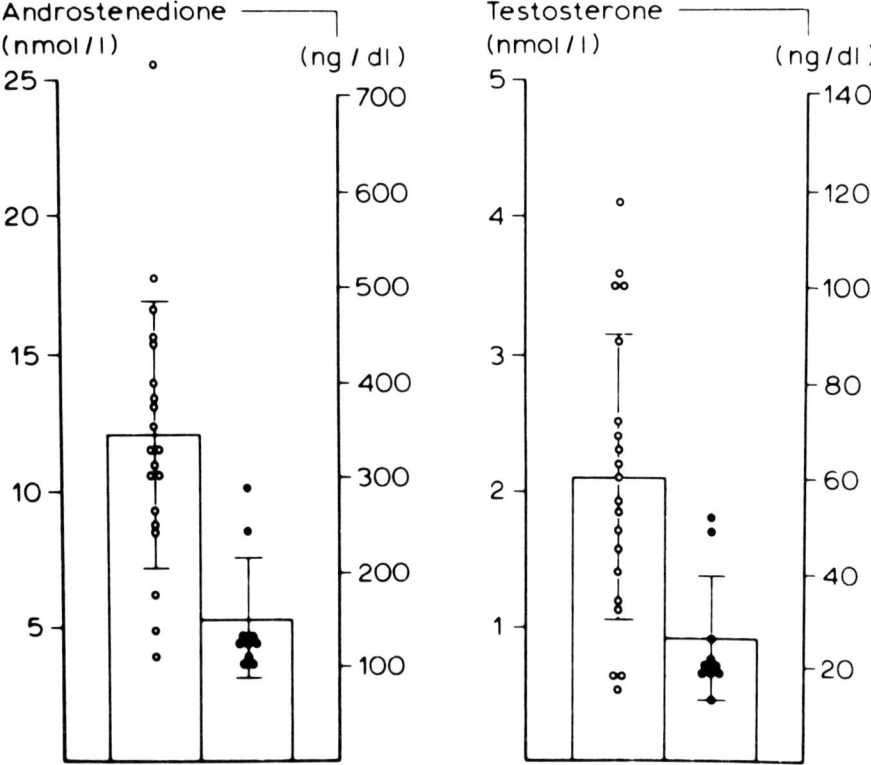

Figure 3 Serum androstenedione and testosterone concentrations in 20 PCO patients (open circles) and ten control women (solid circles)

Table 1 Changes of the LH/FSH ratio in 20 women with the PCO syndrome during 12 weeks of Diane® administration. Blood samples were obtained 7 days after the end of each 3-week medication period

	Periods of Diane® administration		
Changes of the LH/FSH ratio	I	II	III
Increase	7	5	3
Decrease	10	13	15
No change	1	1	0
Missing values	2	1	2

level after withdrawal of medication was significantly lower than the pretreatment concentration ($p = 0.03$) (Figure 5). The estradiol concentration after 2 weeks of ovarian suppression was significantly lower than the pretreatment concentration ($p = 0.003$). Withdrawal of the drug after 3 weeks caused an increase of the estradiol level to pretreatment concentrations.

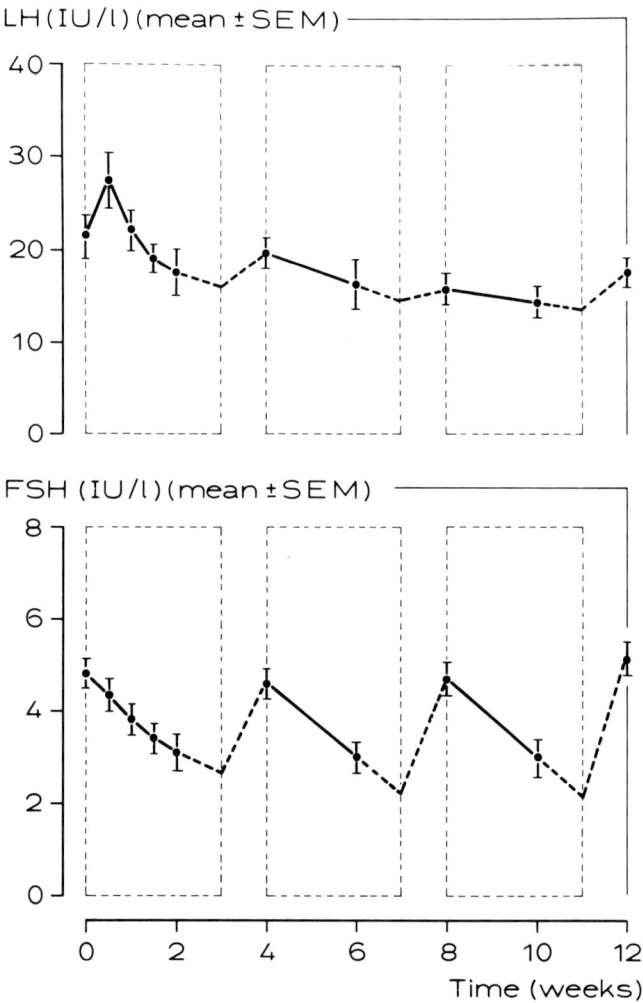

Figure 4 Serum LH and FSH concentrations in the PCO group ($n = 20$) during ovarian suppression (mean $\pm$ SEM). The dotted rectangles indicate the three periods of Diane® treatment. The dotted line indicates the expected trend of increase and decrease of LH and FSH levels in each third week of Diane® administration and each period of medication withdrawal. For changes of the LH/FSH ratio see Table 1

During the next two periods of Diane® administration the same pattern of changes was seen. A rise of estradiol concentrations was demonstrated during the last recovery period (Figure 6). The androstenedione concentrations after 2, 6, 8 and 10 weeks of ovarian suppression were significantly lower

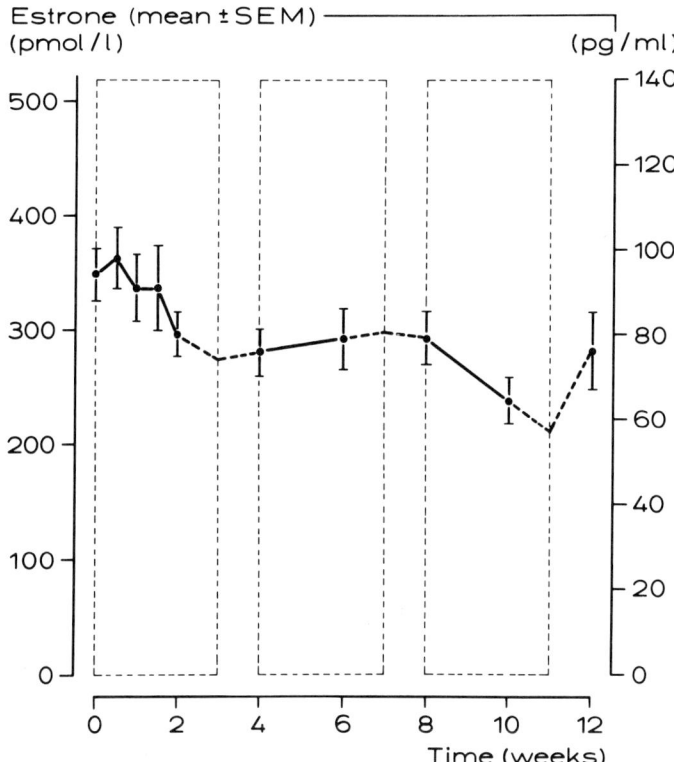

Figure 5 Serum estrone concentrations in the PCO group (*n* = 20) during ovarian suppression (mean ± SEM). The dotted rectangles indicate the three periods of Diane® treatment. The dotted line indicates the expected trend of increase and decrease of estrone levels in each third week of Diane® administration and each period of medication withdrawal

than the pretreatment levels ($p = 0.004$; $p = 0.004$; $p = 0.02$; $p = 0.001$, respectively). At the end of the third recovery period the mean androstene-dione concentration was slightly lower than the pretreatment level ($p = 0.08$) (Figure 7). During the first, second and third period of ovarian suppression a decrease of testosterone levels was seen. During the third period of Diane® administration a significantly reduced testosterone concentration could be demonstrated ($p = 0.01$). A rapid recovery of testosterone levels was seen after the final withdrawal of medication (Figure 8).

Clinical and hormonal data indicated the presence of an ovulatory cycle in five out of 17 PCO patients (29%) who wished to conceive following the period of ovarian suppression. Two women of this group became pregnant in the first spontaneous cycle. Some endocrine details concerning one of these conception cycles are depicted in Figure 9.

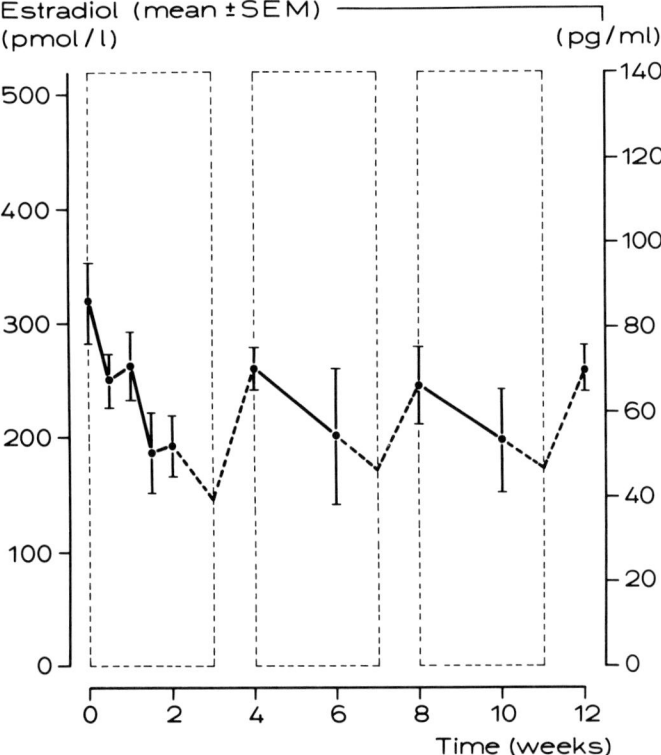

Figure 6 Serum estradiol concentrations in the PCO group ($n = 20$) during ovarian suppression (mean $\pm$ SEM). The dotted rectangles indicate the three periods of Diane® treatment. The dotted line indicates the expected trend of increase and decrease of estradiol levels in each third week of Diane® administration and each period of medication withdrawal

DISCUSSION

The dynamics of gonadotropin and steroid changes in PCO patients, using an estrogen–progestogen combination preparation, were studied. Twenty PCO patients used a combination preparation which contained cyproterone acetate and ethinylestradiol for a period of 12 weeks in a discontinuous way. The LH and FSH levels decreased during the treatment period. After withdrawal of the medication, a rapid increase of FSH levels was seen, whereas the LH concentration remained relatively low. Consequently, the LH/FSH ratio tended to normalize during the recovery period. A decrease of the estrogen (estrone, estradiol) and androgen (androstenedione, testosterone) levels was seen during the use of the combination preparation. After withdrawal of this medication, the estrogen concentrations remained relatively low, whereas the androgen concentrations returned to levels comparable with the pretreatment concentrations.

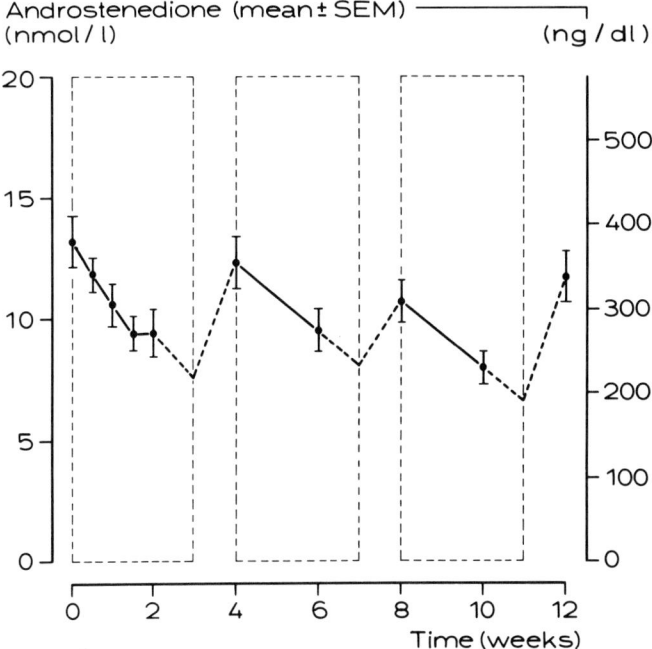

Figure 7 Serum androstenedione concentrations in the PCO group ($n = 20$) during ovarian suppression (mean $\pm$ SEM). The dotted rectangles indicate the three periods of Diane® treatment. The dotted line indicates the expected trend of increase and decrease of androstenedione levels in each third week of Diane® administration and each period of medication withdrawal

In several other studies, the effects of oral contraceptive combination preparations on hormonal and clinical parameters in PCO patients were investigated[7–10]. Estrogen–progestogen combination preparations resulted in the normalization of elevated LH levels and elevated total and unbound testosterone levels. An increase of testosterone binding globulin levels has been reported as well. In a time-course study Raj et al.[7] demonstrated that unbound testosterone declined within a week of initiating treatment with Loestrin® and that by 12–16 weeks the level was completely normal.

From our findings and results reported in the literature one may conclude that, due to the decreased LH/FSH ratio with the concomitantly reduced serum estrogen levels, the conditions for follicular maturation were improved when compared with the pretreatment situation. In order to obtain better conditions for follicular maturation in patients with the PCO syndrome, ovarian suppression with a combination preparation seems justified in women with chronic hyperandrogenic anovulation.

However, in the second part of our study, which concerned some aspects of the process of follicular maturation following the ovarian suppression period, this conclusion could not be established. Only five out of 17 patients ovulated. Since occasional ovulatory cycles may occur spontaneously in

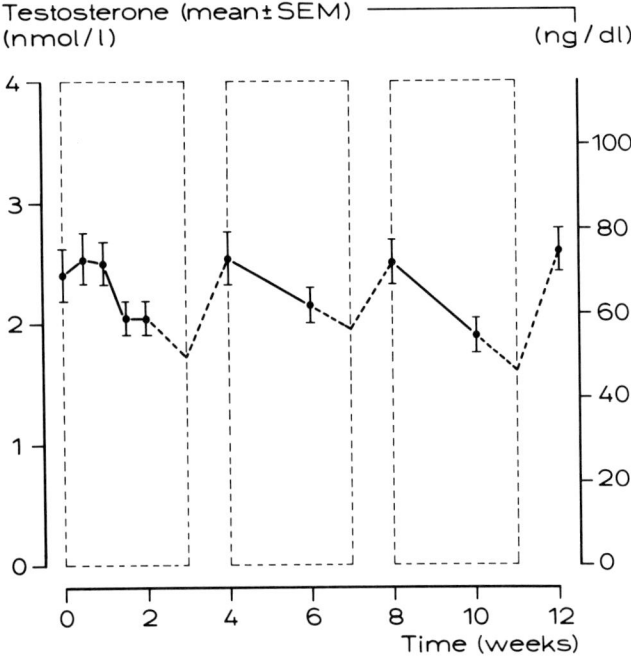

Figure 8 Serum testosterone concentrations in the PCO group ($n = 20$) during ovarian suppression (mean ± SEM). The dotted rectangles indicate the three periods of Diane® treatment. The dotted line indicates the expected trend of increase and decrease of testosterone levels in each third week of Diane® administration and each period of medication withdrawal

women with the PCO syndrome (incidence 20–30% according to Goldzieher and Axelrod[11] and Baird et al.[12]), it is not possible to conclude that ovulation in the present study was in any way related to the preceding period of ovarian suppression. The suppressive effect of oral contraceptive steroids on the hypothalamic–pituitary–ovarian axis in normal women disappears within a few days following discontinuation of the contraceptive preparation. After the initial recovery period, a completely normal endocrine function was found and up to 86% of women ovulated within 6 weeks[13–16]. By comparing these data from the literature with the results of the present study and findings reported by Cullberg[17], who also studied some endocrine aspects of follicular maturation in PCO patients following the use of an oral contraceptive (Marvelon®), it can be seen that inadequate follicular maturation is characteristic for most PCO patients, even after a period of ovarian suppression[18].

Figure 9 Some hormonal changes (following ovarian suppression) in a conception cycle of a PCO patient. Following the period of ovarian suppression, the serum levels of FSH, LH, estradiol, estrone, testosterone and androstenedione were determined. In this figure these values are presented. The mean ± 2SD of the same parameters in the anovulatory group ($n = 12$) are also indicated.

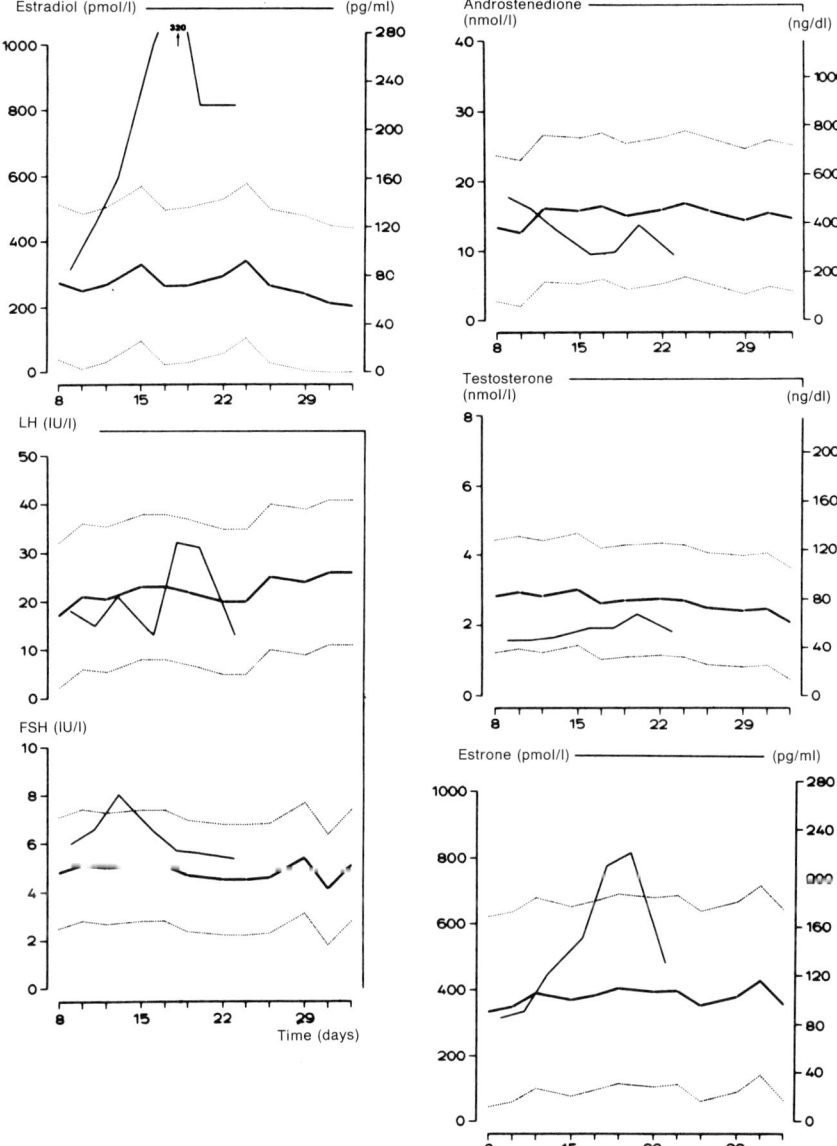

An adequate release of FSH is seen. This FSH release resulted in successful follicular maturation which is reflected by the rise of the estradiol and estrone levels. An LH surge can be seen and ovulation followed. The progesterone concentrations were determined on cycle days 23, 25 and 30; they were 11.0, 20.0 and 32.0 ng/ml, respectively. The testosterone level was rather low in comparison with the mean testosterone concentration of the anovulatory group.

At the onset of this ovulatory cycle the testosterone concentration was fairly normal, whereas the androstenedione level was rather high when compared with androgen concentrations determined in normal ovulatory women during the early follicular phase.

After 11 years of primary infertility, the patient became pregnant during this cycle. At a menstrual age of 28 weeks she delivered a son; this boy is doing well

REFERENCES

1. Stein, I.F. and Leventhal, M.L. (1935). Amenorrhea associated with bilateral polycystic ovaries. *Am. J. Obstet. Gynecol.*, **29**, 181
2. Yen, S.S.C., Chaney, C. and Judd, H.L. (1976). Functional aberrations of the hypothalamic–pituitary system in the polycystic ovary syndrome: a consideration of the pathogenesis. In James, V.H.T., Serio, M. and Giusti, G. (eds.) *The Endocrine Function of the Human Ovary*, pp. 373–85. (London: Academic Press)
3. Burger, C.W., Korsen, T.J.M., Hompes, P.G.A., van Kessel, H. and Schoemaker, J. (1986). Ovulation induction with pulsatile luteinizing releasing hormone in women with clomiphene citrate-resistant polycystic ovary-like disease: clinical results. *Fertil. Steril.*, **46**, 1045
4. Fleming, R. (1988). Induction of ovulation in polycystic ovarian disease patients. *The Releaser*, **3**, 8
5. Zweers, D.J., Evers, J.L.H., Heineman, M.J. and Hamilton, C.J.C.M. (1989). Promising high cumulative pregnancy rate in LHRH analogue/hMG/hCG treated PCO patients. Presented at the *International Symposium on the Present Place of LHRH Analogues in Gynaecology*. June, Brussels, Belgium
6. Heineman, M.J., Thomas, C.M.G., Doesburg, W.H. and Rolland, R. (1984). Hormonal characteristics of women with clinical features of the polycystic ovary syndrome. *Eur. J. Obstet. Gynecol. Reprod. Biol.*, **17**, 263
7. Raj, S.G., Raj, M.H.G., Talbert, L.M., Sloan, C.S. and Hicks, B. (1982). Normalization of testosterone levels using a low estrogen-containing oral contraceptive in women with polycystic ovary syndrome. *Obstet. Gynecol.*, **60**, 15
8. Cullberg, G., Hamberger, L., Mattson, L.A., Mobacken, H. and Samsioe, G. (1985). Effects of low-dose desogestrel-ethinylestradiol combination on hirsutism, androgens and sex hormone binding globulin in women with a polycystic ovary syndrome. *Acta Obstet. Gynecol. Scand.*, **64**, 195
9. Calaf-Alsina, J., Rodriguez-Espinosa, J., Cabero-Roura, A., Lenti-Paoli, O., Mora-Brugues, J. and Estaban-Altirriba, J. (1987). Effects of a cyproterone-containing oral contraceptive on hormonal levels in polycystic ovarian disease. *Obstet. Gynecol.*, **69**, 255
10. Nappi, C., Farace, M.J., Leone, F., Minutolo, M., Tommaselli, A.P. and Montemagno, U. (1987). Effect of a combination of ethinylestradiol and desogestrel in adolescents with oligomenorrhea and ovarian hyperandrogenism. *Eur. J. Obstet. Gynecol. Reprod. Biol.*, **25**, 209
11. Goldzieher, J.W. and Axelrod, L.R. (1963). Clinical and biochemical features of polycystic ovarian disease. *Fertil. Steril.*, **14**, 631
12. Baird, D.T., Corker, C.S., Davidson, D.W., Hunter, W.M., Michie, E.A. and Van Look, P.F.A. (1977). Pituitary–ovarian relationships in polycystic ovary syndrome. *J. Clin. Endocrinol. Metab.*, **45**, 798
13. Loraine, J.A., Bell, E.T., Harkness, R.A., Mears, E. and Jackson, M.C.N. (1965). Hormone excretion patterns during and after the long-term administration of oral contraceptives. *Acta Endocrinol.*, **50**, 15
14. Rice-Wray, E., Correu, S., Gorodovsky, J., Esquivel, J. and Goldzieher, J.W. (1967). Return of ovulation after discontinuance of oral contraceptives. *Fertil. Steril.*, **18**, 212
15. Klein, T.A. and Mishell, D.R. (1977). Gonadotropin, prolactin, and steroid hormone levels after discontinuation of oral contraceptives. *Am. J. Obstet. Gynecol.*, **127**, 585
16. Lahteenmakin, P., Ylostalo, P., Sipinen, S., Toivonen, J., Ruusuvaara, L., Pikkola, P., Nilsson, C.G. and Luukkainen, T. (1980). Return of ovulation after abortion and after discontinuation of oral contraceptives. *Fertil. Steril.*, **34**, 246
17. Cullberg, C. (1985). Pharmacodynamic studies on desogestrel administered alone and in combination with ethinylestradiol. *Acta Obstet. Gynecol. Scand.*, Suppl. 133
18. Heineman, M.J. (1982). *The Polycystic Ovary Syndrome*, Thesis, Nijmegen, The Netherlands

16

The treatment of chronic hyperandrogenemic states: adrenal suppression

T.J. McKenna

INTRODUCTION

Idiopathic hirsutism (IH) and polycystic ovary syndrome (PCOS) are related disorders both associated with chronic hyperandrogenemia[1,2]. The disorders are distinguished by the development of more profound hyperandrogenemia in PCOS and the consequent occurrence of hyperestrogenemia and the characteristic abnormalities in gonadotropin secretion. On rare occasions it is possible to document a specific cause for hyperandrogenemia, e.g. androgen-secreting adrenal tumor[3], congenital adrenal hyperplasia[4], or Cushing's syndrome[5]. However, such an association is relatively rare. In the majority of PCOS patients the precise sequence of events leading to the development of hyperandrogenemia in PCOS is the subject of ongoing debate[2,6,7]. The possibility that a primary abnormality in the adrenal gland may play a fundamental role in the development of PCOS is suggested by a number of related observations. It was noted previously that PCOS may develop secondary to florid and well recognized adrenal abnormalities[3-5]; dehydroepiandrosterone sulfate (DHEAS), the most plentiful steroid normally present in the adult woman, is uniquely of adrenal origin and is found to be elevated in many patients with PCOS[8]. Furthermore, when rats were treated with adrenal androgens, they developed ovarian abnormalities analogous to PCOS[9]. Prompted by these observations, we have examined adrenal function in patients with IH and PCOS by comparing glucocorticoid and androgen responses to stimulation with exogenous α1–24-adrenocorticotropic hormone (ACTH) and to endogenous stimulation in response to metyrapone. Metyrapone inhibits 11β-hydroxylase and thereby impairs the final step in cortisol biosynthesis. As a result of this, plasma cortisol levels fall and ACTH and related pro-opiomelanocortin fragments are secreted in an attempt to overcome the block in cortisol biosynthesis[10]. However, stimulated adrenal androgen biosynthesis is not perturbed by exhibition of metyrapone. In addition, the plasma concentration of the cortisol precursor, 11-deoxycortisol, can be used as an index of activity in the cortisol biosynthetic pathway.

Patients with IH demonstrated elevated testosterone, testosterone/sex hormone binding globulin ratios (an index of free testosterone), dihydrotestosterone, androstenedione and 17-hydroxyprogesterone levels. The androstenedione, dehydroepiandrosterone (DHEA), and 17-hydroxyprogesterone increments, following stimulation with ACTH, 250 μg intramuscularly, were significantly higher than increments occurring in normal women (Table 1). Furthermore, 8 h following the administration of metyrapone, the testosterone increment in plasma of women with IH was significantly higher than that occurring in normal women[11]. When the metyrapone-induced plasma steroid responses were examined in PCOS patients, the increments achieved in testosterone, androstenedione and 11-deoxycortisol were excessive (Table 1)[12]. These observations indicate the presence of adrenal hyperresponsiveness in both androgen and glucocorticoid pathways in patients with IH or PCOS. The pattern achieved does not conform to any of the classical enzymatic defects occurring in congenital adrenal hyperplasia[13]. Although 17-hydroxyprogesterone increments following ACTH were higher than in normal women, the levels achieved were much lower than those seen in patients with 21-hydroxylase deficiency. When plotted on the nomogram described by New and co-workers[13], the levels achieved fall within the range described for the general population. The possibility of Cushing's syndrome had been excluded in all subjects using the overnight dexamethasone suppression test[14]. The question then addressed was could the steroid abnormalities be corrected by adrenal suppression and, if so, what effect would this have on gonadotropin secretion and ovarian function in PCOS?

ADRENAL SUPPRESSION

Dexamethasone, 0.5 mg given each night on retiring, was chosen as the treatment option to attempt long-term adrenal suppression. We have previously demonstrated that this treatment is effective in inducing regular ovulation in women with classical 21-hydroxylase deficiency[15]. Furthermore,

Table 1 Incremental steroid responses (nmol/l, mean ± SD) to ACTH and metyrapone in idiopathic hirsutism (IH) and polycystic ovary syndrome (PCOS)

	PCOS/IH untreated	PCOS/IH Dex-treated	Normal women untreated
ACTH[11]			
Androstenedione	4.5 ± 3.8*	1.2 ± 1.3†	2.0 ± 1.5
DHEA	39 ± 23*	15 ± 13†	18 ± 25
17-hydroxyprogesterone	3.2 ± 1.8*	2.3 ± 2.5	1.8 ± 1.1
Cortisol	511 ± 329*	473 ± 255*	252 ± 122
Metyrapone[12]			
Testosterone	1.5 ± 0.6*	0.6 ± 0.6†	1.1 ± 0.4
Androstenedione	16.2 ± 5.7*	8.4 ± 90†	10.8 ± 3.0
11-Deoxycortisol	453 ± 136*	192 ± 130*†	353 ± 101

*Significantly different from normal women, $p < 0.05$; †significantly different from untreated PCOS/IH, $p < 0.05$; ‡ dexamethasone-treated

this low dosage treatment is equivalent to physiological glucocorticoid requirement and thus avoids the criticism of potentially suppressing gonado-tropin secretion directly as a result of a pharmacological effect. Whereas glucocorticoid excess was associated with suppression of gonadotropin secretion[16], dexamethasone 0.5 mg each night supported the occurrence of ovulation in congenital adrenal hyperplasia[15]. Evaluation of the response to treatment was undertaken 3–6 months after the start of dexamethasone administration; however, on the evening when metyrapone was administered, dexamethasone was omitted.

Following treatment with dexamethasone, previously elevated testosterone and androstenedione levels were similar to those occurring in normal women; the testosterone to sex hormone binding globulin ratio was significantly suppressed while sex hormone binding globulin levels rose significantly (Table 2). In addition, DHEA and DHEAS levels were suppressed to values significantly lower than those seen in normal women[11,12]. The mean estrone level fell in women with PCOS following treatment with dexamethasone but was still significantly higher than that seen in normal women. Basal luteinizing hormone (LH) levels were similar prior to and following treatment with dexamethasone in PCOS. The maximum LH increment induced by luteinizing hormone releasing hormone (LHRH), 200 μg i.v., which was significantly higher in PCOS than in normal women prior to treatment, was no longer significantly different following treatment; however, the mean level achieved was still higher than that seen in normal women (Table 2).

The excessive testosterone and androstenedione responsiveness to metyr-apone seen in PCOS was markedly suppressed following treatment with dexamethasone so that the increments noted were significantly lower than those seen in untreated normal women (Table 1)[12]. While the mean 11-deoxycortisol response to metyrapone was suppressed following treatment with dexamethasone, 12 of 16 patients maintained a normal glucocorticoid response[17]. This observation is important when considering the possibility of glucocorticoid excess during treatment, or of adrenal suppression following the withdrawal of dexamethasone. Indeed, the excessive cortisol response to ACTH persisted following treatment with dexamethasone in IH[11]. This suggests that an adrenal abnormality persisted following suppression of adrenal stimulation (Table 1).

Table 2 The hormonal response to dexamethasone in PCOS

	PCOS untreated	PCOS treated	Normal women untreated
Testosterone (nmol/l)	1.9 ± 0.7*	1.4 ± 0.7	1.3 ± 0.4
Testosterone/sex hormone binding globulin ratio	9.0 ± 6.8*	4.8 ± 2.6*†	3.1 ± 1.3
Androstenedione (nmol/l)	9.8 ± 3.3*	6.6 ± 3.5†	6.0 ± 1.8
Estrone (pmol/l)	293 ± 136*	237 ± 109*	177 ± 70
Maximum LH response to LHRH (mIU/l)	47 ± 39*	38 ± 45	13 ± 12

* Significantly different from normal women, $p < 0.05$; † significantly different from untreated PCOS, $p < 0.05$

145

In our original study, ten of 15 patients who were submitted to extensive evaluation resumed regular ovulatory menstrual bleeding. In a much more extensive clinical experience, the response rate of approximately two-thirds of patients has been maintained. Approximately 50% of patients, in whom ovulation is induced using dexamethasone treatment, continue to ovulate regularly when the dose of dexamethasone is reduced to 0.25 mg each night. Approximately 50% of patients, treated with dexamethasone for 6 months, demonstrate improvement in hirsutism[11]. Occasional patients, particularly those who are significantly overweight at the initiation of treatment, tend to gain significantly more weight when taking dexamethasone. Only very rarely do patients complain of gastrointestinal upset or depression on the dosage used.

DISCUSSION

The rationale for use of adrenal suppression in the treatment of PCOS has been developed in this report, i.e. the presence of hyperandrogenemia associated with adrenal glucocorticoid and androgen hyperresponsiveness to exogenous and endogenous stimulation. Therefore, it is appealing to speculate that subtle adrenal abnormalities may be primary to the development of PCOS in the usual patient where a distinct primary diagnosis cannot be made. In the present paper we summarize the results obtained when chronic adrenal suppression was undertaken using non-pharmacological doses of dexamethasone. Dexamethasone was administered at night only to blunt the early morning surge in ACTH and related peptides which occurs prior to waking[17]. Dexamethasone is ideal for this purpose because of its prolonged biological half-life. We have previously demonstrated that this dosage schedule of dexamethasone was associated simultaneously with the resolution of signs of glucocorticoid excess which had occurred and the control of congenital adrenal hyperplasia which had not been achieved using cortisone acetate 37.5 mg per day in divided doses[18]. Successful treatment of patients with PCOS with dexamethasone was associated with significant suppression of testosterone and testosterone/sex hormone binding globulin ratios, which was not seen in patients who failed to respond[12]. However, there was a fall in the mean estrone levels amongst responders but a small increase in those of non-responders. The responsiveness of both testosterone and androstenedione to metyrapone was significantly suppressed in responders but not in the clinical non-responders. While both clinical groups demonstrated suppression of 11-deoxycortisol responsiveness to metyrapone, this was much more profound in responders than in non-responders. Poor compliance of non-responders to treatment with dexamethasone is one possible explanation for these differences[12].

The frequency of establishing regular ovulation induced by continued treatment with dexamethasone is similar to the rate of achieving a single ovulation induced by the necessarily intermittent administration of clomiphene citrate[19,20]. In contrast, clomiphene citrate may be associated with the occurrence of hyperstimulation syndrome, which is never seen in patients treated with dexamethasone. Furthermore, while clomiphene citrate may induce transient hyperandrogenemia, dexamethasone is associated with suppression of androgens. It is likely that, while clomiphene citrate alters acutely abnormal gonadotropin secretion and specifically reverses FSH suppression transiently, treatment with dexamethasone probably reverses in an ongoing manner a more fundamental abnormality in the pathogenesis of PCOS[2]. Thus, the suppression of androgen levels with dexamethasone was associated with a lowering of estrone levels and a lessening of abnormality in gonadotropin levels (Table 1).

The present discussion has not addressed the problem of hirsutism frequently seen in patients with PCOS. During prolonged treatment with dexamethasone, for at least 6 months, approximately 50% of patients exhibit both a subjective and an objective reduction in the number of hairs present, the rate of hair regrowth and the frequency with which cosmetic measures are required. With more prolonged use the improvement in hirsutism, particularly facial, increases and this is frequently associated with clearance of coexisting acne.

Adrenal suppression with dexamethasone in low dose provides an ideal form of treatment for approximately 60–70% of patients with PCOS. This form of treatment tends to be under-used, probably because at least 3 months of treatment is necessary before the full impact on the syndrome can be assessed. The opportunity to promptly ascertain the outcome of intervention, i.e. in approximately 3 weeks, appears to have rendered clomiphene citrate more popular. The end results of inducing ovulation and pregnancy appear to be similar with the two forms of treatment. However, dexamethasone has advantages, particularly in women who wish to establish regular ovulation on an ongoing basis while not desiring to become pregnant at that time. There is compelling clinical experience to indicate that early treatment will render fertility more likely when it is subsequently desired. Treatment for 1–2 years with dexamethasone 0.25–0.5 mg each night is frequently associated with continued normal ovulatory function following the cessation of the treatment.

REFERENCES

1. McKenna, T.J., Cunningham, S.K. and Loughlin, T. (1985). The adrenal cortex and virilization. *Clin. Endocrinol. Metab.*, **14**, 997–1020
2. McKenna, T.J. (1988). Pathogenesis and treatment of polycystic ovary syndrome. *N. Engl. J. Med.*, **318**, 558–62
3. Kase, E.N., Kowal, J., Perloff, W. and Soffer, L.J. (1963). *In vitro* production of androgens by virilizing adenoma and associated polycystic ovaries. *Acta Endocrinol.*, **44**, 15–19
4. Hague, W.M., Honour, J.W., Adam, J., Vecsei, P. and Jacobs, H.S. (1989). Steroid responses to ACTH in women with polycystic ovaries. *Clin. Endocrinol.*, **30**, 355–66
5. Yen, S.S.C. (1980). Polycystic ovary syndrome. *Clin. Endocrinol.*, **12**, 177–207
6. Barnes, R. and Rosenfeld, R.L. (1989). The polycystic ovary syndrome: pathogenesis and treatment. *Ann. Intern. Med.*, **110**, 386–99
7. Stewart, P.M., Shackleton, C.H.L., Beastall, T.H. and Edwards, C.R.W. (1990). 5α-reductase activity in polycystic ovary syndrome. *Lancet*, **335**, 431–3

8. Hoffman, D.I., Klove, K. and Lobo, R.A. (1984). Prevalence and significance of elevated dehydroepiandrosterone sulphate levels in anovulatory women. *Fertil. Steril.*, **42**, 76–81

9. Mahesh, V.B. (1983). Various concepts of pathogenesis of polycystic ovary disease. In Mahesh, V.B. and Greenblatt, R.B. (eds.) *Hirsutism and Virilization, Pathogenesis, Diagnosis and Management*, pp. 247–76. (Boston: John Wright)

10. Cunningham, S.K., Loughlin, T., Bertagna, X., Girard, F. and McKenna, T.J. (1988). Plasma pro-opiomelanocortin fragments and adrenal steroids following administration of metyrapone in normal and hirsute women. *J. Endocr. Invest.*, **11**, 247–53

11. Moore, A., Magee, F., Cunningham, S., Culliton, M. and McKenna, T.J. (1983). Adrenal abnormalities in idiopathic hirsutism. *Clin. Endocrinol.*, **18**, 391–9

12. Loughlin, T., Cunningham, S., Moore, A., Culliton, M., Smyth, P.P.A. and McKenna, T.J. (1986). Adrenal abnormalities in polycystic ovary syndrome. *J. Clin. Endocrinol. Metab.*, **62**, 142–7

13. White, P.C., New, M.I. and Dupont, B. (1987). Congenital adrenal hyperplasia. *N. Engl. J. Med.*, **316**, 1519–24, 1580–6

14. Cronin, C., Igoe, D., Duffy, M.J., Cunningham, S.K. and McKenna, T.J. (1990). The overnight dexamethasone test is a worthwhile screening procedure. *Clin. Endocrinol.*, **33**, 27–33

15. McKenna, T.J., Moore, G., Orth, D.N., Burr, I.M., Liddle, G.W. and Lacroix, A. (1980). The biosynthesis of androgens in 21-hydroxylase deficiency. In Genazzani, A.R., Thijssen, J.H.H. and Siiteri, P.K. (eds.) *Adrenal Androgens*, pp. 135–9. (New York: Raven Press)

16. Sakakura, M., Takebe, K. and Nakagawa, S. (1975). Inhibition of luteinizing hormone secretion induced by synthetic LRH by long-term treatment with glucocorticoids in human subjects. *J. Clin. Endocrinol. Metab.*, **40**, 774–9

17. Cunningham, S.K., Moore, A. and McKenna, T.J. (1983). Normal cortisol response to corticotropin in patients with secondary adrenal failure. *Arch. Intern. Med.*, **143**, 2276–9

18. Moore, G., Lacroix, A., Rabin, D. and McKenna, T.J. (1980). Gonadal dysfunction in adult men with congenital adrenal hyperplasia. *Acta Endocrinol.*, **95**, 185–95

19. Gorlitsky, G.A., Kase, N.G. and Speroff, L. (1978). Ovulation and pregnancy rates with clomiphene citrate. *Obstet. Gynecol.*, **51**, 265–9

20. Gysler, M., March, C.M. and Mishell, D.R. Jr. (1982). A decade's experience with individualized clomiphene treatment regime including its effect on the post-coital test. *Fertil. Steril.*, **37**, 161–7

17

Antiandrogens in polycystic ovary syndrome

G. Schaison

Hyperandrogenism is one of the characteristic endocrine abnormalities of the polycystic ovary syndrome (PCOS). Some cryptic cases may have no skin changes. However, acne, seborrhea and a masculine pattern of hirsutism are usually prominent features which are also influenced by racial factors. In more severe cases, hair loss and clitoromegaly may occur. In almost all cases, women with PCOS call for effective treatment of their hirsutism.

The ovary is the major source of androgen excess as demonstrated by direct measurement of androgen production in adrenal and ovarian venous samples[1]. In PCOS, the increased luteinizing hormone (LH) secretion is the main cause of androgen hypersecretion[2]. The production rate of androgens of ovarian origin is constantly elevated. The increase of plasma androstenedione is one of the characteristics of the disease. Total plasma testosterone levels may be normal but plasma free or non-sex hormone binding globulin (SHBG) bound testosterone is very often increased. Indeed, SHBG concentrations are almost always subnormal in PCOS. It was generally accepted that the androgen/estrogen balance was the mediator of the reduction in SHBG. More recently, it has been demonstrated that obesity, hyperinsulinemia and growth factors directly affect SHBG concentrations[3].

Plasma or urinary 3α-androstenediol glucuronide is increased in PCOS. This conjugated androgen metabolite reflects accurately the 5α-reductase activity at the receptor level and should be constantly elevated in hirsute women[4].

The possibility that adrenal androgens may be involved in some cases cannot be definitively excluded[5]. Dehydroepiandrosterone sulfate (DHEAS) of almost exclusive adrenal origin has been found to be increased in some patients. Regulation of DHEAS is independent of pituitary–ovarian function. The administration of a potent long-acting gonadotropin releasing hormone (GnRH) agonist completely suppresses plasma androstenedione and testosterone levels but does not modify DHEAS levels. In women with PCOS, a late onset of 3β-hydroxysteroid dehydrogenase deficiency was previously claimed to be the cause of increased plasma DHEAS levels. However, the most recent studies did not confirm this hypothesis[6].

On the other hand, hyperinsulinemia observed in both obese and non-obese patients may contribute to the androgen hyperproduction[7]. Insulin resistance, sometimes associated with acanthosis nigricans, has been reported to be a common finding in PCOS[8,9]. Insulin may exert its effect on ovarian stroma through an interaction with the insulin-like growth factor 1 receptors[10].

Finally, hyperandrogenism may play a role in the pathophysiology of the syndrome. Androgens directly or through aromatization to estrogens may be responsible for the distortion in gonadotropin secretion. Many conditions involving androgen excess simulate PCOS. In female to male transsexual subjects, long-term administration of high doses of testosterone may, directly at the ovarian level, induce follicular atresia and polycystic ovary syndrome-like histopathological changes[11].

Correcting ovarian overproduction of androgens is one of the therapeutical goals in PCOS. Before starting therapy, the patients should understand that results of treatment cannot be expected before 6–12 months due to the cyclic activity of the hair follicles, which varies from one anatomical region to another. It is also important to emphasize the fact that PCOS is a life-long disorder for which caloric restriction and weight loss must be included in the overall approach and are mandatory to optimize treatment.

Contraceptive pills were the first line of treatment to inhibit gonadotropin secretion and suppress hyperandrogenism. However, the C-19 progestin contained in these pills limited their indication. The recent contraceptive pills with the new generation of non-androgenic 19-nortestosterone derivatives are a good alternative for treatment even though the antigonadotropic effect is less potent.

Suppression of androgen production can also be achieved through inhibition of androgen biosynthesis or gonadotropin inhibition by GnRH analogs.

The antifungal drug, ketoconazole, is an inhibitor of cytochrome P-450-dependent enzymes in various organs. Thus, this compound inhibits the adrenal and ovarian synthesis of androgens, but it also blocks glucocorticoid synthesis which prevents its use in the treatment of hirsutism in PCOS.

GnRH agonists in women with PCOS have been proposed. We have used a long-acting depot preparation of GnRH agonist[12]. Biocompatible and biodegradable microcapsules containing and releasing 100 μg per day of D-Trp[6]-GnRH in a 30-day period were administered intramuscularly once a month for 3 months. After a transient flare-up, there was a complete suppression of the LH response to GnRH following 1 week of treatment. After a transient increase, there was a dramatic decrease to castration levels of plasma estradiol, estrone, androstenedione and testosterone levels by the second week of treatment. Marked clinical improvement and normalization of ovarian size were obtained. However, basal and stimulated gonadotropin levels and ovarian steroid levels returned to pretreatment values 3 months after the last injection of the agonist. These data suggest that, whatever the pathophysiology of this syndrome, it remains a permanent situation. The once-a-month use of microcapsules of GnRH agonist is practical, convenient and should improve patient compliance. However, long-term use of this drug alone with its potential problems of medical castration – hot flushes, vaginal dryness and osteoporosis – is not advised. However, the association of the agonist with progesterone and 17β-estradiol will normalize the ovaries and correct the hyperandrogenism while maintaining hormonal equilibrium.

Inhibition of androgen can be achieved by 5α-reductase inhibitors or true antiandrogens acting directly on the androgen receptor in the target tissue.

Antiandrogens acting at the receptor level can be divided into two classes, steroidal or non-steroidal. Steroidal antiandrogens are estrogens, progestins and spironolactone. Estrogens have an antigonadotropic action and increase SHBG concentrations. Some progestins are potent steroid antiandrogens. Chlormadinone acetate and megestrol acetate interact with the progesterone receptor and have a strong antigonadotropic activity.

Cyproterone acetate (CPA) is a synthetic 17-hydroxyprogesterone derivative with both antiandrogen and antigonadotropic activities. In women with PCOS, it is the most effective drug, which corrects the hyperandrogenism by suppressing ovarian androgen secretion and by inhibiting peripheral androgen action. It has been used in combination with estrogens as a contraceptive for many years. In women with PCOS, this treatment corrects the hyperandrogenism by inhibiting peripheral androgen action and by suppressing ovarian androgen secretion. As a progestin, cyproterone acetate prevents endometrial hyperplasia caused by unopposed estrogen exposure. Its long half-life (38 h) allows once-daily administration. The drug is administered at a dose of 50 mg/day for 20 days. It accumulates in fatty tissues and its elimination is so prolonged that a reverse sequential regime has been advised. 17β-estradiol, administered orally or percutaneously, may be used in association with cyproterone acetate in case of contraindications to ethinylestradiol[13].

In ten women with PCOS, we compared[12] the efficacy of CPA and GnRH D-Trp[6]-GnRH. CPA was given in daily doses of 50 mg for 3 months. Basal plasma LH levels decreased significantly and the LH response to GnRH was also reduced but not abolished (Figure 1). CPA suppressed gonadotropin secretion less completely than did GnRH agonist. Ovarian suppression was also less profound than after D-Trp[6] GnRH. However, plasma testosterone levels were below 0.5 ng/ml (1.7 nmol/l) and plasma androstenedione below 1 ng/ml (3.5 nmol/l) (Figure 2). It is noteworthy that urinary 3α-diol glucuronide remained elevated. This may be explained by the action of CPA which is a non-specific inducer of hepatic enzymes. Likewise, mean plasma SHBG concentration, already low in patients with PCOS, further decreased after CPA administration. The mechanism by which CPA decreases plasma SHBG levels remains unknown. However, this action cannot be explained by an androgen agonist effect of CPA.

It has been reported that CPA interacts with the glucocorticoid receptors and has a partial glucocorticoid activity. However, administered in normal women, 200 mg of CPA for 6 days did not decrease the cortisol and the ACTH response to ovine corticotropin releasing hormone (CRH) (Figure 3). Thus its glucocorticoid activity is certainly negligible when the dose is lower than 100 mg/day.

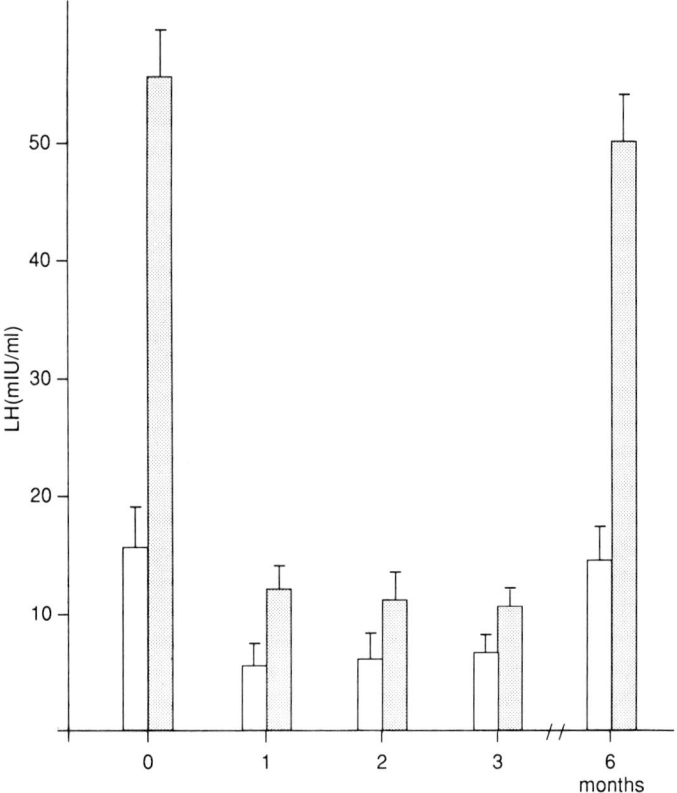

Figure 1 Effects of CPA on mean ($\pm$ SEM) GnRH-stimulated plasma LH levels on day 5 of each month of treatment in ten PCO patients

No side-effects were reported by any of the patients during treatment with CPA alone. Transient uterine bleeding caused by the progestational properties of the drug occurred in some patients. However, intermittent CPA administration in combination with estrogens prevents this side-effect. Breast tenderness, decrease of libido and vaginal dryness were unusual. However, despite the 1200 calories/day direct, body weight did not change during CPA treatment. CPA has no effect on carbohydrate and lipid metabolism but obesity may be a contraindication to this treatment.

CPA is not available in the United States. Thus, spironolactone is currently used. It diminishes testosterone biosynthesis by decreasing the microsomal cytochrome P-450 content (17-hydroxylase and 17–20 desmolase). The antiandrogen effect is also exerted through inhibition of dihydrotestosterone binding to the androgen receptor. However, its metabolite, canrenone, has a very weak affinity for the androgen receptor. It is administered in a dose of 100 mg daily for 21 days with a 7-day break in treatment. In our opinion, this therapy has a weak antiandrogenic activity.

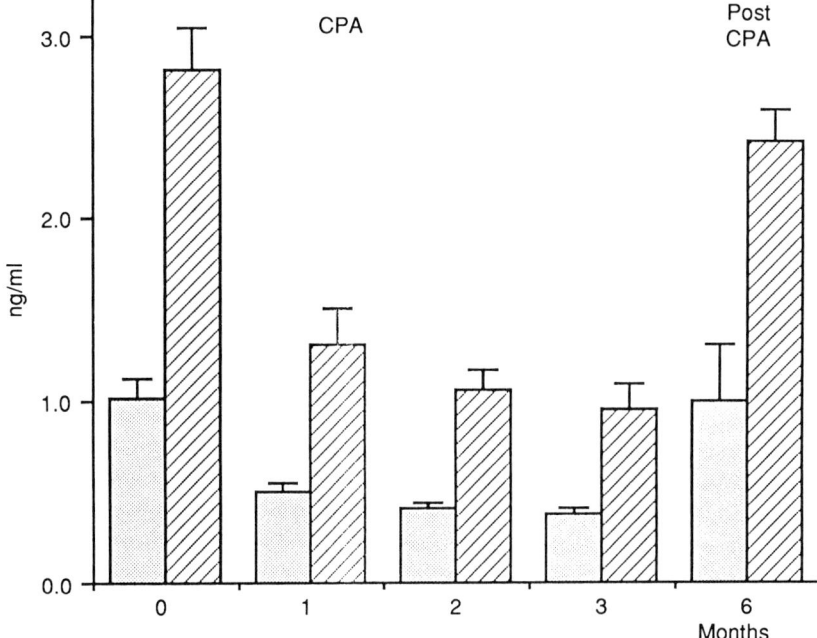

Figure 2 Mean ($\pm$ SEM) plasma androstenedione (hatched bars) and testosterone (solid bars) concentrations in ten PCO patients during treatment with CPA and 3 months after discontinuation of therapy (to convert plasma androstenedione and testosterone to nmol/l, multiply by 3.492 and 3.467, respectively)

Non-steroidal antiandrogens are pure antiandrogens. All are devoid of antigonadotropic activity and must be associated with a contraceptive method. Cimetidine has a very low affinity for the androgen receptor and is not really effective. Flutamide needs to be converted into hydroxyflutamide *in vivo* to exert its antiandrogenic activity. Side-effects are hepatotoxicity and gastrointestinal troubles. It has not been extensively studied in women with PCOS. However, at a dose of 500 mg in combination with an oral contraceptive, it is highly effective on the hyperandrogenism.

We used another non-steroidal antiandrogen, Anandron (5,5-dimethyl 3-4-nitro-3 (trifluoromethyl) phenyl 2,4 imidazolinedione), which interacts only with the androgen receptor. It has no androgen, progestin or antigonadotropic effects and has a half-life of 48 h[14]. Its affinity for the androgen receptor is 100 times less than testosterone itself and its properties are similar to those of flutamide.

We used this new and pure antiandrogen as a tool to study the effect of androgen suppression on the hypothalamo–pituitary axis in nine patients with PCOS[15]. They received Anandron 100 mg twice daily and placebo in a cross-over design study for 2 consecutive months separated by 1 month. LH pulse frequency and amplitude were studied by sampling every 10 min

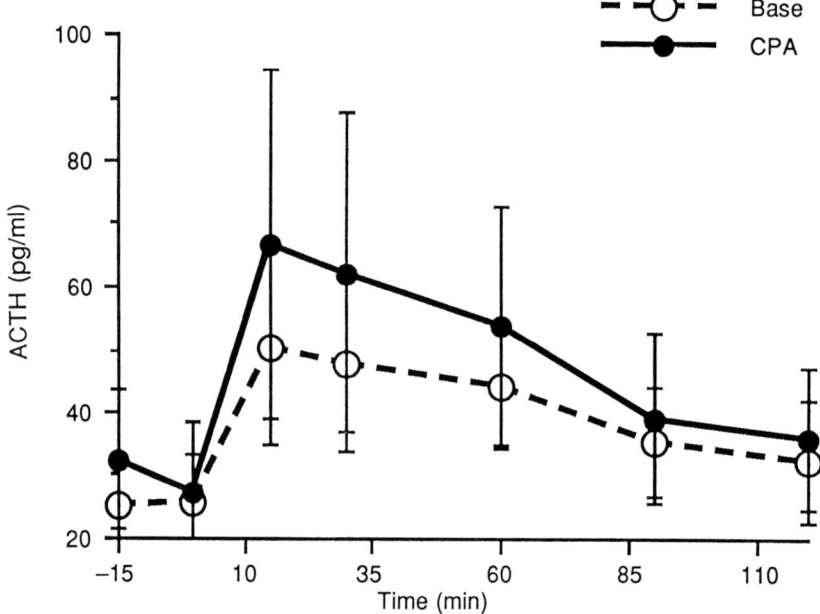

Figure 3 ACTH response to CRH on day 6 of CPA administration in normal women (to convert to pmol/l multiply by 0.22)

for 8 h and analyzed by cluster analysis. The LH response to GnRH was determined on day 5 of each month. Plasma androstenedione, SHBG and urinary 3α-diol glucuronide were measured on days 5, 10, 20 and 24 of each month. Short-term treatment with Anandron did not change the LH pulsatile profile (Figure 4) nor the LH response to GnRH, demonstrating that androgens, apart from their aromatization to estrogens, do not directly play a role in the distortion of gonadotropin secretion in PCOS.

Plasma androstenedione levels were not modified (Figure 5). SHBG did not change significantly. As an antiandrogen, Anandron should have decreased the 5α-reductase activity. However, 3α-diol glucuronide did not change after 2 months of treatment. Clinically, there was no significant change in ovarian volume at the end of the study but acne, seborrhea and hirsutism, in the following months, were dramatically improved. No side-effects were observed. However, interstitial pneumonia, gastrointestinal trouble, impaired visual adaptation to darkness and intolerance to alcohol have been reported in men with prostatic carcinoma treated with high doses of Anandron and these must be considered.

A well-tolerated non-steroidal antiandrogen in combination with oral contraceptives may be, in the future, a highly effective therapy for hirsutism in polycystic ovarian disease.

5α-Reductase inhibitors such as 4-azasteroid are currently under clinical trials in men with benign prostatic hypertrophy[16]. They have no affinity for the androgen receptor, no estrogenic, progestational or gonadotropin-

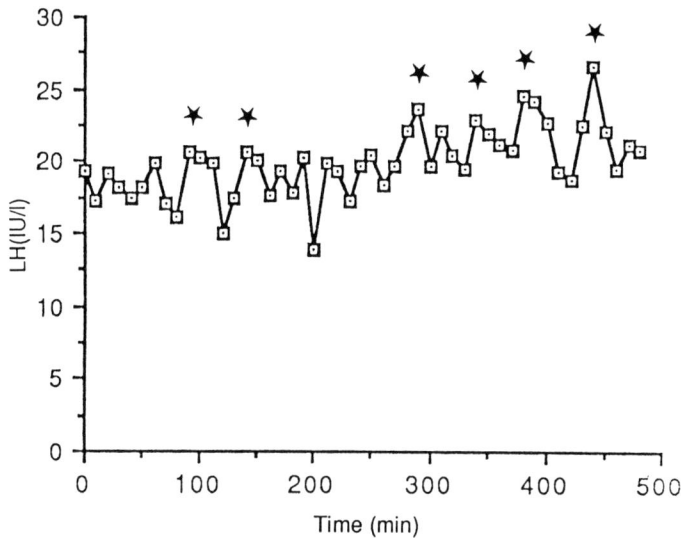

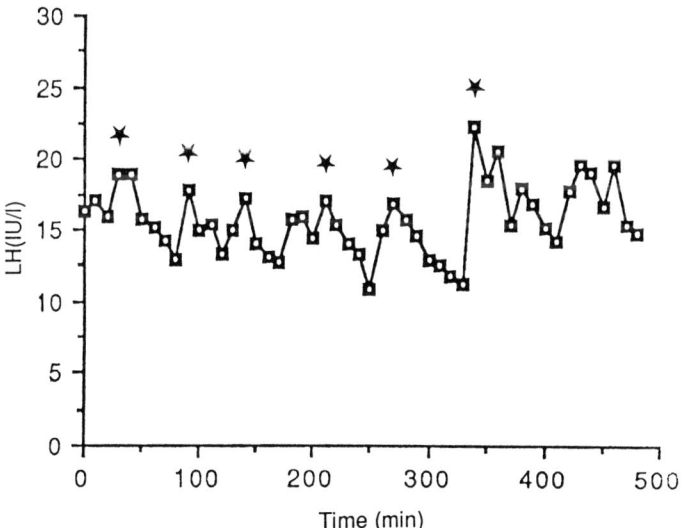

(a)

Figure 4 Pulsatile LH profile from one patient with PCOS on day 5 of each month of Anandron (a) or placebo (b) treatment. The asterisks indicate significant pulses

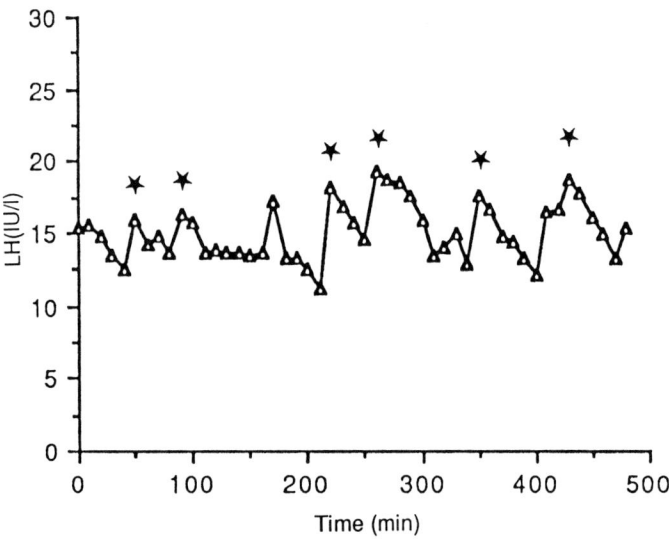

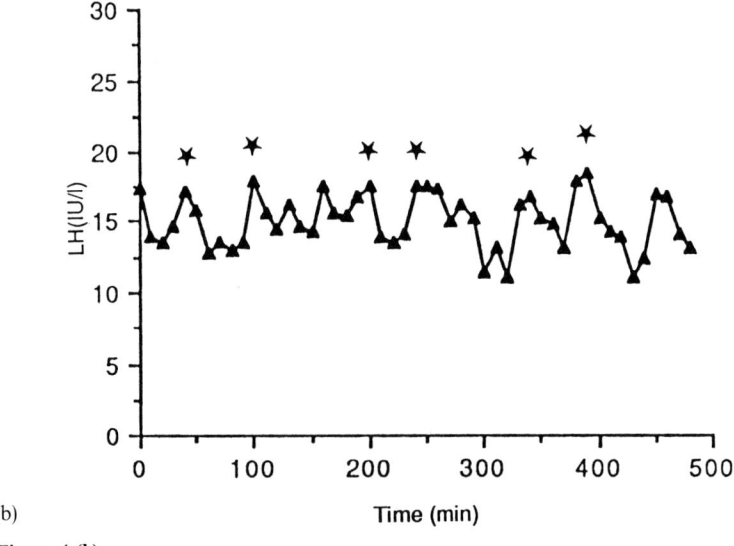

(b)

Figure 4 (b)

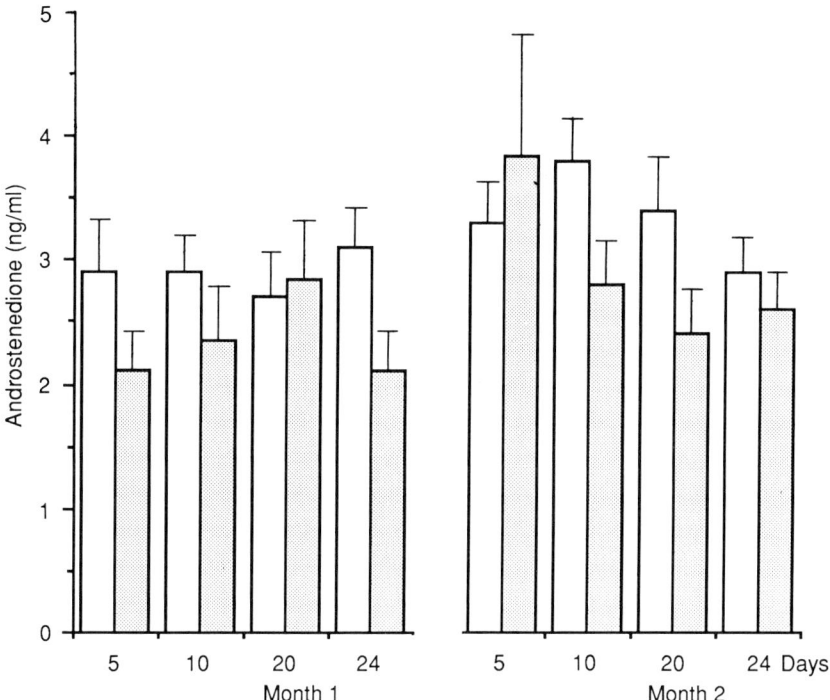

Figure 5 Mean ($\pm$ SEM) plasma androstenedione levels in nine women with PCOS on days 5, 10, 20 and 24 of Anandron (empty bars) or placebo (solid bars) treatment

inhibiting potency. Moreover, they have no side-effects. They have not yet been used in women but it is expected that, in the near future, they will be tested in association with gonadotropin inhibition in the treatment of hirsutism in women with PCOS.

It is also important to take cosmetic approaches into account. Bleaching may be all that is needed in mild cases. Electrolysis by a trained technician is the only permanent means of hair removal but is expensive and often tedious. Nevertheless, it is a useful adjunct after 4–6 months of antiandrogen treatment.

ACKNOWLEDGEMENTS

The expert assistance of Dr B. Couzinet and the secretarial support of Mrs G. Lanvier are gratefully acknowledged.

REFERENCES

1. Kirschner, M.A. and Jacobs, J.B. (1971). Combined ovarian and adrenal vein catheterization to determine the site(s) of androgen over-production in hirsute women. *J. Clin. Endocrinol. Metab.*, **33**, 199–209
2. Kazer, R.R., Kessel, B. and Yen, S.S. (1987). Circulating luteinizing hormone pulse frequency in women with polycystic ovary syndrome. *J. Clin. Endocrinol. Metab.*, **65**, 233–6
3. Glass, A.R., Swerdloff, R.S., Bray, G.A., Dahma, W.T. and Atkinson, R.C. (1977). Low serum testosterone and sex hormone binding globulin in massively obese men. *J. Clin. Endocrinol. Metab.*, **45**, 1211–15
4. Horton, R., Hawks, D. and Lobo, R. (1982). 3α 17β androstanediol glucuronide in plasma: a marker of androgen action in idiopathic hirsutism. *J. Clin. Invest.*, **69**, 1203–6
5. McKenna, T.J. (1988). Pathogenesis and treatment of polycystic ovary syndrome. *N. Engl. J. Med.*, **318**, 558–62
6. Barnes, R. and Rosenfield, R. (1989). The polycystic ovary syndrome: pathogenesis and treatment. *Ann. Intern. Med.*, **110**, 386–99
7. Burghen, G.A., Givens, J.R. and Kitabashi, A.E. (1980). Correlation of hyperandrogenism with hyperinsulinism in polycystic ovary disease. *J. Clin. Endocrinol. Metab.*, **50**, 113–16
8. Dunaif, A., Graf, M., Mandeli, J., Laumas, V. and Dobrjansky, A. (1987). Characterization of groups of hyperandrogenic women with acanthosis nigricans, impaired glucose tolerance, and/or hyperinsulinemia. *J. Clin. Endocrinol. Metab.*, **65**, 499–507
9. Dunaif, A. (1986). Do androgens directly regulate gonadotropin secretion in the polycystic ovary syndrome? *J. Clin. Endocrinol. Metab.*, **63**, 215–21
10. Adashi, E.Y., Resnick, C.E., D'Ercole, A.J., Svoboda, M.E. and van Wyk, J.J. (1985). Insulin-like growth factors as intraovarian regulators of granulosa cell growth and function. *Endocr. Rev.*, **6**, 400–20
11. Sinder, T., Spijkstra, J.J., Van der Tweel, J.G., Burger, C.W., Van Kessel, H., Hompes, P.G.A. and Gooren, L.J.G. (1989). The effects of long term testosterone administration on pulsatile luteinizing hormone secretion and on ovarian histology in eugonadal female to male transsexual subjects. *J. Clin. Endocrinol. Metab.*, **69**, 151–7
12. Couzinet, B., Le Strat, N., Brailly, S. and Schaison, G. (1986). Comparative effects of cyproterone acetate or a long acting gonadotropin releasing hormone agonist in polycystic ovarian disease. *J. Clin. Endocrinol. Metab.*, **63**, 1031–5
13. Kuttenn, F., Rigaud, C., Wright, F. and Mauvais-Jarvis, P. (1980). Treatment of hirsutism by oral cyproterone acetate and percutaneous estradiol. *J. Clin. Endocrinol. Metab.*, **51**, 1107–11
14. Raynaud, J.P., Bonne, C., Bouton, M.M., Lagace, L. and Labrie, F. (1979). Action of a non-steroid anti-androgen, RU 23906, in peripheral and central tissues. *J. Steroid. Biochem.*, **11**, 93–9
15. Couzinet, B., Thomas, G., Thalabard, J.C., Brailly, S. and Schaison, G. (1989). Effects of a pure antiandrogen on gonadotropin secretion in normal women and in polycystic ovarian disease. *Fertil. Steril.*, **52**, 42–50
16. Brooks, J.R. (1986). Treatment of hirsutism with 5α-reductase inhibitors. In Horton, R. and Lobo, R.A. (eds.) *Clinics in Endocrinology and Metabolism, Androgen Metabolism in Hirsute and Normal Females*, pp. 293–306. (London, Philadelphia and Toronto: W.B. Saunders)

18

Endocrine changes after ovarian surgery in patients with polycystic ovary syndrome

H.J. van Geldorp

INTRODUCTION

Even with the use of increasing doses of clomiphene citrate (CC) with or without the addition of human chorionic gonadotropin (hCG), 10–15% of women with polycystic ovary syndrome (PCOS) remain anovulatory[1]. Parenteral treatment with human menopausal gonadotropin (hMG) and hCG or pure follicle stimulating hormone (FSH) under careful hormonal and ultrasound monitoring can induce ovulatory cycles. The alternative treatment, by ovarian wedge resection, as found by Stein and Leventhal[2], and the endocrine responses to this treatment studied by hormone measurements in blood samples and described by several authors[3-5], has largely been abandoned because of the need for laparotomy and the potential for development of pelvic adhesions[6,7].

Microsurgical techniques for ovarian wedge resection can prevent adhesion formation and have brought new life to this treatment. This study was proposed to evaluate the clinical and hormonal response to microsurgical wedge resection of the ovaries in a selected group of women with PCOS who failed to ovulate with CC and hCG. The serum levels of testosterone, androstenedione, estradiol, FSH and luteinizing hormone (LH) before and after the microsurgical wedge resection were examined. The results are compared with those described recently for less extensive surgical techniques involving laparoscopic ovarian cautery or laser vaporization[8-13].

MATERIAL AND METHODS

Sixteen women between the ages of 22 and 36 years with clinical and biochemical findings of PCOS were studied. All women had anovulatory cycles and failed to ovulate on 150–200 mg CC daily for 5 days with or without hCG (5000–10 000 IU). The other criteria for inclusion were the following: primary infertility, elevated serum LH levels and low-to-normal FSH levels, with at least an LH/FSH ratio of 2:1; normal serum levels of prolactin and dihydroepiandrostenedione sulfate (DHEAS).

In all women a first-look laparoscopy was performed to exclude other factors that could interfere with fertility such as tubal pathology or severe adhesions. All ovaries showed signs of PCOS: a smooth, white surface and containing multiple small subcapsular cysts. No therapy was given between the day of laparoscopy and laparotomy, in general a period of 3 months. Laparotomy was performed by a Pfannenstiel-incision and, if there were some thin adhesions, they were removed carefully with a unipolar electric needle. The wedge resection was performed with this needle and the stroma of the ovary was sutured with 3 x 0 atraumatic Vicryl, followed by inverted suturing of the cortex with 6 x 0 Prolene (non-absorbable). After careful cleaning of the abdominal cavity with Ringers solution enriched with heparin, the abdominal wall was closed as usual in a 4-layer method followed by the skin with an intracutaneous Prolene 3 x 0 suture.

The women were studied before and after operation to assess serum levels of the following hormones: LH, FSH, estradiol, androstenedione, testosterone and progesterone. Blood samples were drawn 1 day before operation, 1 day after the operation, at 6 weeks, 3 months and then monthly until 6 months after the operation. All hormone determinations were made in the follicular phase of the cycle. In seven women a pregnancy was achieved within 6 months; these patients were excluded from further hormonal follow-up. Serum progesterone and testosterone levels were determined by radioimmunoassay techniques as described previously[14,15]. LH and FSH were measured by double-antibody radioimmunoassay with materials obtained from UCB (Braine-l'Alleud, Belgium), using preparations MRC 68/40 and 69/104 as standards, respectively. Concentrations of androstenedione were estimated by radioimmunoassay using kits provided by Diagnostic Products Corporation, Los Angeles, USA. Normal values were: testosterone, 0.7–3.0 nmol/l; LH (follicular phase), 1.0–8.0 IU/l; androstenedione, 3–12 nmol/l; FSH (follicular phase), 1.2–4.2 IU/l; estradiol, 75–370 pmol/l (follicular phase). A serum progesterone level of at least 13 nmol/l was considered as a strong indication that ovulation had occurred.

RESULTS

There were no complications from the treatment and all patients were discharged home within 7 days. Fourteen patients ovulated and menses occurred between 24 and 36 days after operation. Seven became pregnant within 6 months and were excluded from further follow-up. Additional treatment with CC was given after the first 6 months in nine patients and three of them became pregnant within another 6 months. Three women were ovulating regularly on a dosage of 50 mg CC and one on a dosage of 100 mg CC, but these three women did not conceive within the 6 months of additional therapy. Two patients did not ovulate after the operation during the whole study period. The serum concentrations of LH, FSH, estradiol, testosterone and androstenedione of the nine patients that did not conceive within the first 6 months after the operation are summarized in Table 1.

Table 1 Concentrations (mean $\pm$ SEM) of hormones the day before the operation and at times after the operation ($n = 9$)

	LH (IU/l)	FSH (IU/l)	Estradiol (pmol/l)	Andro- stenedione (nmol/l)	Testo- sterone (nmol/l)
Day -1	16.4 ± 2.1	4.6 ± 0.6	204 ± 13	18.24 ± 2.12	4.9 ± 0.4
Day 1	11.6 ± 2.5	7.4 ± 0.8	109 ± 24	15.47 ± 1.42	3.6 ± 0.3
Week 6	13.0 ± 4.1	3.6 ± 0.7	254 ± 29	10.20 ± 1.37	3.1 ± 0.4
Month 3	9.8 ± 1.1	4.3 ± 0.6	486 ± 84	11.83 ± 1.79	3.5 ± 0.3
Month 4	8.2 ± 2.7	4.0 ± 0.2	492 ± 78	12.34 ± 1.67	3.4 ± 0.4
Month 5	8.9 ± 4.1	3.7 ± 0.5	467 ± 101	12.87 ± 1.91	3.7 ± 0.2
Month 6	7.8 ± 1.6	4.3 ± 0.3	510 ± 43	13.62 ± 1.47	3.5 ± 0.4

Serum concentrations of androstenedione (Figure 1) and testosterone (Figure 2) decreased after operation and no remarkable differences were observed between the seven pregnant patients and those not pregnant within 6 months. Serum concentrations of LH, FSH and estradiol of the nine non-conceiving patients in the first 6 months after the operation are shown in Figure 3.

After the operation, a fall in the serum LH level from 16.4 ± 2.1 IU/l before operation to 11.6 ± 2.5 IU/l 1 day after the operation and further to almost normal levels was seen in contrast to the FSH levels that showed an increase in the immediate postoperative period followed by a decrease after the 3rd month. Preoperative values of estradiol were 204 ± 13 pmol/l, falling to 109 ± 24 pmol/l, followed by an increase to high normal levels in the following months. The rapid fall in androgen levels after the operation is dramatic and precedes changes in the other hormones. No significant differences were observed in the serum concentrations of androstenedione, testosterone and estradiol between the two non-responders to ovarian surgery and those who ovulated after the procedure, but no decrease in the serum LH level was observed and the postoperative rise in FSH showed a slower pattern than in the other patients.

DISCUSSION

The spontaneous occurrence of ovulation and pregnancy in patients with PCOS is well recognized and the syndrome is known to be unpredictable. But it seems clear that even without controls the occurrence of ovulation in 14 out of 16 patients (87%) with chronic anovulation immediately after microsurgical ovarian wedge resection is more than coincidental. The results of this therapy can be easily compared to reported ovulation rates for CC therapy with response rates of 67–76% or hMG–hCG treatment with a successful induction of ovulation in 75–95%[1] of cases, but also to alternative means of ovulation by laparoscopic electrocautery and laser vaporization with ovulation rates of 72–92%[8-13] and 71%, respectively in the first postoperative weeks.

Earlier reports of the incidence of successful ovulation after ovarian wedge

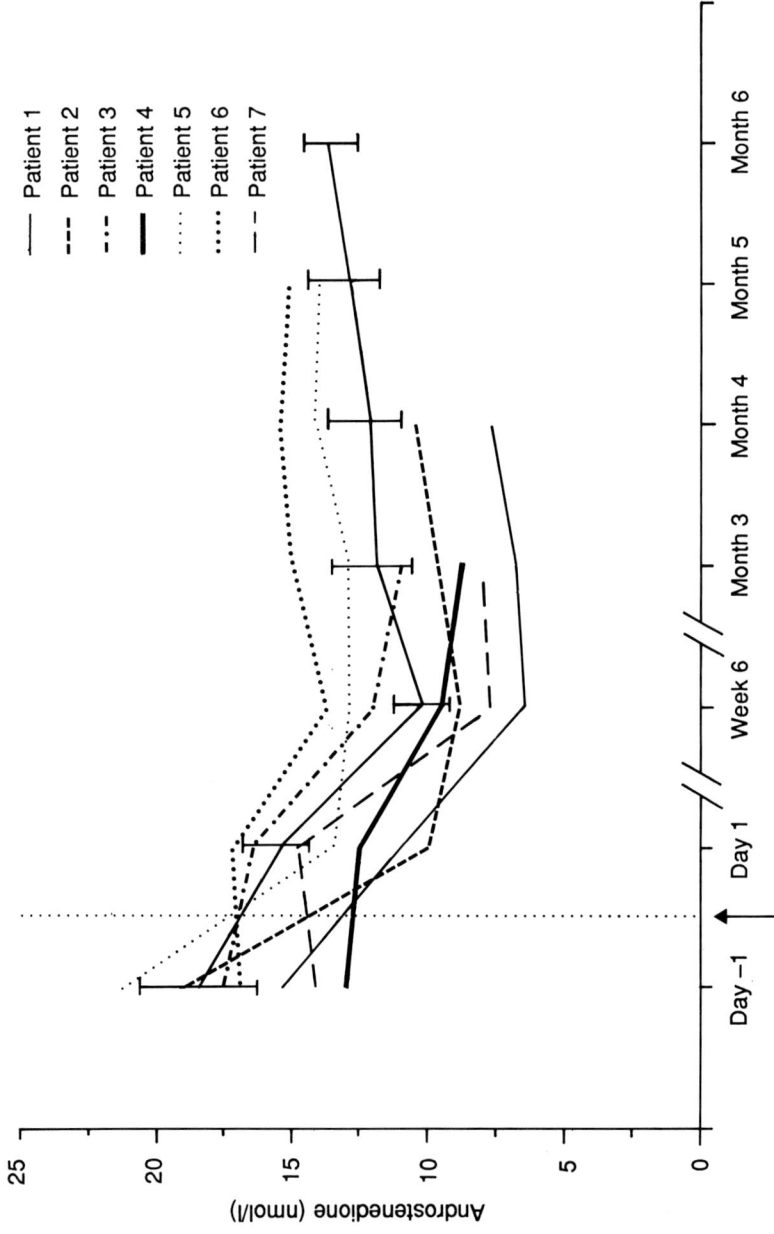

Figure 1 Androstenedione concentrations (nmol/l) in seven pregnant patients and in patients not pregnant after 6 months (mean ± SEM)

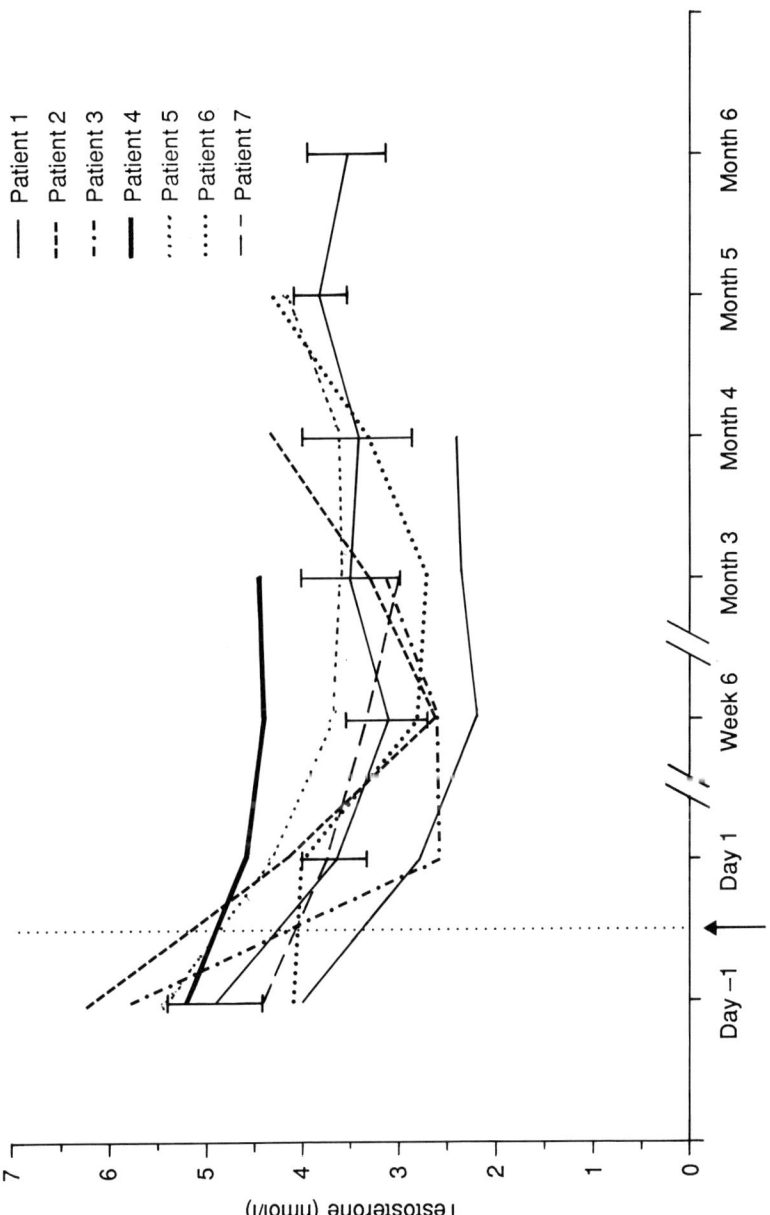

Figure 2 Testosterone concentrations (nmol/l) in seven pregnant patients and in patients not pregnant after 6 months (mean ± SEM)

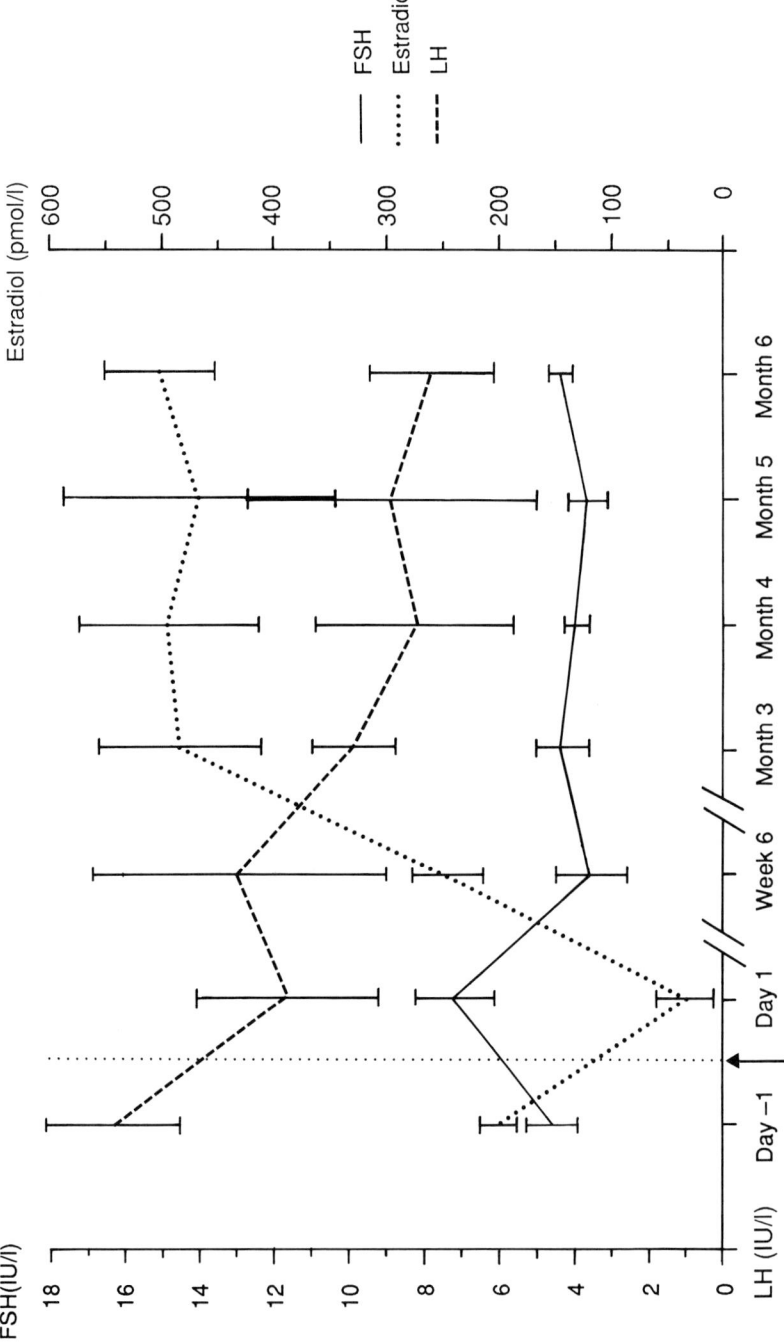

Figure 3 LH, FSH and estradiol concentrations in nine non-conceiving patients in the first 6 months after the operation (mean ± SEM)

resection vary quite widely in the literature with a mean of 80%[16]. The mechanism by which ovarian wedge resection induces ovulation is still unknown. The explanation, that the mechanical barrier to ovulation was removed by incision of the thickened ovarian capsule[2], is too simplistic and several investigators have studied the hormonal alterations associated with ovarian wedge resection in an attempt to determine the mechanism of action[4,5]. The almost consistent finding in these studies is a dramatic fall in serum androgen levels in the first days of the postoperative period. Judd and co-workers studied eight patients with PCOS undergoing wedge resection and suggested that the decreased androgen levels may have removed an intraovarian block to follicular maturation or that the hyperemia associated with postoperative inflammation allowed increased delivery of gonadotropins[4]. Katz and co-workers[5], in a study of two patients, theorized that the postoperative decreases in estradiol and androgens eliminate a persistent positive feedback effect of these steroids on the pituitary. The LH levels return to normal and the normalization of FSH/LH ratio then allows follicular maturation to proceed. Gjönnaess[8] postulated that laparoscopic ovarian cautery destroyed the inhibiting principal ('dominant') follicle and thus allowed ovulation to occur. Daniell and Miller[13] suggested that another possibility may be that, by physically opening the capsular cysts with the laser, the follicular fluid that contains androgens is removed from the ovarian environment and subsequently suctioned out of the peritoneal cavity at laparoscopy. This may temporarily lower the overall androgen content of the ovaries and thus temporarily resolve the block to ovulation known to be associated with high intraovarian androgen levels. In the present study, we have demonstrated that microsurgical ovarian wedge resection is characterized by a postoperative decrease in androstenedione and testosterone as well as a decrease in LH and estradiol, together with an increase in FSH in the first few weeks after the operation. These results have recently also been described in alternative means of treatment such as laparoscopic cautery[9–12] and laser vaporization[13], but the period of postoperative hormonal changes seems much longer in microsurgical wedge resection and the tendency to return to preoperative values and anovulation much lower. This microsurgical treatment of PCOS is, along with laparoscopic treatment, almost certainly only a temporary respite, since the basic physiological disorder is not changed. It is expected that, as time passes, these patients will lapse back into anovulation and even amenorrhea. However, this probably temporary correction of anovulation allows these selected patients to attempt and possibly achieve pregnancy. Further careful evaluation of this renewed operative procedure is needed, with longer follow-up to assess the best operative treatment in severe cases of PCOS.

REFERENCES

1. Frank, S., Adams, J., Mason, H. and Polson, D. (1985). Ovulatory disorders in women with polycystic ovary syndrome. *Clin. Obstet. Gynecol.*, **12**, 605
2. Stein, I.F. and Leventhal, H.I. (1935). Amenorrhea associated with bilateral polycystic

ovaries. *Am. J. Obstet. Gynecol.*, **29**, 181

3. Lloyd, C.W., Lobotsky, J., Segre, E.J., Kobayaski, T., Taymor, M.L. and Batt, R.E. (1966). Plasma testosterone and urinary 17-ketosteroids in women with hirsutism and polycystic ovaries. *J. Chir. Endocrinol. Metab.*, **26**, 314
4. Judd, H.L., Riggs, L.A., Anderson, D.C. and Yen, S.S.C. (1976). The effects of ovarian wedge resection in circulating gonadotropin and ovarian steroid levels in patients with polycystic ovary syndrome. *J. Clin. Endocrinol. Metab.*, **43**, 347
5. Katz, M., Carr, P.J., Cohen, B.M. and Millow, R.W. (1978). Hormonal effects of wedge resection in polycystic ovaries. *Obstet. Gynecol.*, **51**, 437
6. Buttram, V. and Vaguero, C. (1975). Postovarian wedge resection adhesive disease. *Fertil. Steril.*, **26**, 874
7. Eddy, C.A., Asch, R.H. and Balmaceda, J.P. (1980). Pelvic adhesions following microsurgical and macrosurgical wedge resection of the ovaries. *Fertil. Steril.*, **33**, 537
8. Gjönnaess, H. (1984). Polycystic ovarian syndrome treated by ovarian electrocautery through the laparoscope. *Fertil. Steril.*, **41**, 20
9. Asborn, A. and Gjönnaess, H. (1985). Hormonal response to electrocautery of the ovary in patients with polycystic ovary disease. *Br. J. Obstet. Gynecol.*, **92**, 1258
10. Gjönnaess, H. and Norman, N. (1987). Endocrine changes after laparoscopic ovarian cautery in polycystic ovarian syndrome. *Am. J. Obstet. Gynecol.*, **94**, 779
11. Greenblatt, E. and Caspar, R.F. (1987). Endocrine changes after laparoscopic ovarian cautery in polycystic ovarian syndrome. *Am. J. Obstet. Gynecol.*, **156**, 279
12. Sumioki, H., Utsunomyiya, T., Matsuora, K., Korenaga, M. and Kadota, T. (1988). The effect of laparoscopic multiple punch resection of the ovary on hypothalamo–pituitary axis in polycystic ovary syndrome. *Fertil. Steril.*, **50**, 567
13. Daniell, J.F. and Miller, W. (1989). Polycystic ovaries treated by laparoscopic laser vaporization. *Fertil. Steril.*, **51**, 232
14. De Jong, F.H., Baird, D.T. and Van der Molen, H.J. (1974). Ovarian secretion rates of estrogen, androgens and progesterone in normal women and in women with persistent ovarian follicles. *Acta Endocrinol.*, **74**, 575
15. Verjans, H.L., Cooke, B.A., De Jong, F.H., De Jong, C.C. and Van der Molen, H.J. (1973). Evaluation of a radioimmunoassay for testosterone estimation. *J. Steroid Biochem.*, **4**, 665
16. Goldzieher, J.W. and Green, J.A. (1962). The polycystic ovary. Clinical and histological features. *J. Clin. Endocrinol. Metab.*, **22**, 325

SECTION 3

Gynecological problems in chronic hyperandrogenic anovulation

19

Early pregnancy loss in chronic hyperandrogenic anovulation

M.A.H.M. Wiegerinck

INTRODUCTION

The interrelationship between early pregnancy loss and chronic hyperandrogenic anovulation (CHA) is difficult to assess because of the lack of uniform definitions. Early pregnancy loss is a common and time-related phenomenon in human reproduction. About 60% of conceptions fail to continue beyond the date of the expected menstrual period with ovopathology as the main cause[1]. The early pregnancy loss rate is strongly influenced by the method used to define pregnancy. For example, an early pregnancy loss rate of 33%, when pregnancy is defined at 28 days of the cycle, drops to 14% of all pregnancies confirmed after a 2-week menstrual delay[1]. The spontaneous abortion rate of known pregnancies is 10–15% but, depending on maternal age, this figure may increase to 27%[2]. Polycystic ovaries may be a finding in normal ovulatory women and may not be, as a rule, associated with infertility[3]. Women with CHA constitute a more specific category in which the achievement of pregnancy is a major problem. Spontaneous ovulation and subsequent pregnancy will, by definition, be rare events in CHA. To restore ovulation, medical or surgical interventions are needed.

About 50% of women with CHA who wish to have a child will eventually become pregnant in long-term treatment regimens of ovulation-inducing drugs or after surgical procedures[4–7].

OOCYTE QUALITY AND MICROENVIRONMENT

Possible causes of early pregnancy loss in CHA are listed in Table 1. There is no evidence of an intrinsic oocyte defect in CHA. The concept of intrinsically normal oocytes would gain support if complete reversal of the CHA condition resulted in normal fertilization and abortion rates. This still has to be established. The fact that 82% of habitual abortion patients have been shown to have polycystic ovaries[8] does not indicate a relationship with defective oocytes. Endogenous and exogenous factors affecting the timing of fertilization do play a significant role. Delayed fertilization is associated with

Table 1 Possible causes of fetal loss in CHA

Poor oocyte quality	
Influence of the microenvironment	
paracrine factors	
follicular fluid:	oocyte, luteal function
peritoneal fluid:	fertilization, embryo
tubal:	embryonic development
endometrial:	implantation
Effect of drugs in CHA treatment	
direct:	oocyte toxic, teratogenic, luteal phase inadequacy
indirect:	multiple pregnancy, ovarian hyperstimulation syndrome

a marked increase in chromosomal aberrations and subsequent embryonic loss[9]. Endocrine and paracrine stromal factors have been incriminated in playing a role in this respect. A proposed mechanism is an inhibiting function of luteinizing hormone (LH) on oocyte maturation inhibitor, which prevents the completion of the first meiotic division. A high LH level in the follicular phase would permit premature oocyte maturation, resulting in poor fertilization and poor embryo implantation[10]. The steroidal intrafollicular microenvironment reflects the stage of oocyte maturation. High androgen levels are the normal microenvironment of oocytes in the germinal vesicle stage, shifting to an increase in estradiol and progesterone in metaphase I and metaphase II follicles[11]. The androgen levels in hyperstimulated follicles of anovulatory women do not differ from those of normal ovulatory women. In anovulatory women a lower follicular fluid progesterone to estradiol ratio was reported, correlating with impaired maturity and lower fertilizability[12]. Clearly the hyperandrogenic peripheral steroid concentrations do not correlate with follicular fluid concentrations. Whether there is an alteration in other environmental conditions, such as in peritoneal fluid, tubal secretions or endometrial receptivity in CHA patients, is not known. The observation of a lack of peritoneal fluid at laparoscopy in CHA patients with classical polycystic ovaries has been made many times. Since macrophages in peritoneal fluid stimulate the progesterone production of granulosa cells[13], changes in the composition of peritoneal fluid may influence luteal function.

THE EFFECT OF MEDICAL AND SURGICAL INTERVENTION

Surgical treatment aims at the resumption of spontaneous ovulation after the treatment. Ovarian wedge resection or laparoscopic ovarian electrocautery will not have a direct adverse effect on pregnancy outcome. The drugs administered to induce ovulation in CHA patients may exert an effect on the early pregnancy loss ratio in two ways, first by increasing the multiple pregnancy rate with an inherent higher abortion rate. The ovarian hyperstimulation syndrome is a known risk factor of ovulation induction in CHA and higher pregnancy loss rate with this condition is assumed, but not demonstrated. Second, a direct toxic effect of the drugs on oocytes, the process of meiosis, luteal function or endometrial receptivity may occur.

Drugs involved in ovulation induction treatment in CHA are clomiphene, human menopausal gonadotropin (hMG), human chorionic gonadotropin (hCG), 'pure' follicle stimulating hormone (FSH), gonadotropin releasing hormone at pulse intervals (GnRH) and dexamethasone (DEX). High doses of clomiphene compromise the oocyte quality in rats[14]. Whether clomiphene administration is associated with a higher incidence of fetal malformations is disputed; certainly no causal relationship has been established. Clomiphene may induce a defective luteal phase[15]. An increased rate of cytogenetic defects has been observed in oocytes when 20–68 ampules of hMG were administered per cycle (43%) compared with less than 20 ampules (25%)[16]. This finding does not necessarily implicate a toxic effect of hMG. The higher dose of hMG needed to obtain an adequate response may be an indication of a decreased oocyte quality. GnRH analogs with gonadotropin stimulation treatment increase the number of recovered oocytes but not the mean number of embryos capable of developing[17]. The embryo quality has been reported to be poorer with the use of GnRH analogs, but the overall pregnancy outcome is better since the uterine receptivity is improved after GnRH administration[18]. To my knowledge, there are no reports on adverse effects of pulsatile GnRH administration on oocytes or embryo development. A combination of reported pregnancy and abortion rates with various regimens of medication is shown in Table 2. A similar compilation with surgical intervention methods in CHA is presented in Table 3.

Table 2 CHA medication: reported pregnancy and abortion rates

Medication	Ref.	Number of patients	Pregnant		Abortion	
			n	%	n	%
CC	21	220	56	23	21	37
	15	35	30	29	4	40
	7	25	15	60	4	27
hMG–hCG	22	41	29	66	7	29
FSH–hCG	6	18	9	50	2	22
GnRH-A–hMG–hCG	23	34	27	81	—	—
GnRH-A–FSH–hCG	24	9	4	44	1	25
Pulsatile LHRH	25	11	3	27	3	60
	4	54	27	50	9	33
Medication + IVF	26	18	6	33	—	—

Table 3 CHA surgical procedures: reported pregnancy and abortion rates

Surgery	Number of patients	Pregnant		Abortion	
		n	%	n	%
Wedge resection[5]	90	43	49	9	21
Laparoscopic ovarian electrocautery[27]	190	89	47	13	15

FETAL PROTECTION FROM MATERNAL HYPERANDROGENEMIA

Once pregnancy is achieved in CHA women, elevated androgen levels in maternal blood may cause concern for the fetus. Virilization of the female fetus as a consequence of excessive maternal androgens is extremely rare with a single case report on polycystic ovaries of the mother as the source[19]. Fetal protection from virilization when exposed to elevated maternal androgens is provided by a variation in maternal, placental and fetal functions[20]. Increased sex hormone binding globulins in pregnancy decrease the amount of exposure of free testosterone in end organs. Steroid aromatization in the placenta converts androstenedione to estrone and 16-hydroxytestosterone to estriol, thereby reducing the androstenedione and testosterone levels in cord blood. As fetal tissue does not possess sulfatase activity, dehydroepiandrosterone sulfate produced by the fetal adrenals cannot be converted to androgens.

CONCLUSIONS

Women with chronic hyperandrogenic anovulation have major problems in achieving pregnancy. A variety of medical and surgical treatment procedures do result in about 50% of these women becoming pregnant and less than 50% give birth to a child. Early pregnancy loss and chronic hyperandrogenic anovulation are ill defined, which makes a quantification of their interrelationship difficult. The reported abortion rates of various modes of treatment fluctuate around 25%, higher than in a normal fertile population but similar to the abortion rate in assisted procreation techniques for infertile couples.

Women with chronic hyperandrogenic anovulation have endocrine and stromal paracrine factors which probably interfere with gamete synchrony, resulting in a higher proportion of oocyte abnormalities, less efficient fertilization and embryonic loss. A reduction of early pregnancy by the use of GnRH analogs in chronic hyperandrogenic anovulation treatment is as yet speculative. Oocyte development is not hampered by high intrafollicular androgen levels which are normal in a certain phase. Peritoneal fluid, tubal and endometrial factors in chronic hyperandrogenic anovulation might have an influence on oocyte development and luteal function. The induction of multiple pregnancies by medication for chronic hyperandrogenic anovulation will increase the early pregnancy loss rate. Finally, in cases of pregnancy with high serum androgen levels in mothers with chronic hyperandrogenic anovulation, the risk of virilization for the fetus is reduced by maternal, placental and fetal protective mechanisms.

REFERENCES

1. Exalto, N. and Rolland, R. (1985). Gamete quality and fertility regulations. In Rolland, R. *et al.* (eds.) *The Nature of Pregnancy Wastage*, pp. 303–11. (Amsterdam: Elsevier Science Publishers)
2. Gilmore, D.H. and McNay, M.B. (1985). Spontaneous fetal loss rate in early pregnancy. *Lancet*, **1**, 107
3. Polson, D.W., Wadsworth, J., Adams, J. and Franks, S. (1988). Polycystic ovaries – a common finding in normal women. *Lancet*, **1**, 870–2
4. Homburg, R., Armar, N.A., Eshel, A., Adams, J. and Jacobs, H.S. (1988). Influence of serum luteinizing hormone concentrations on ovulation, conception, and early pregnancy loss in polycystic ovary syndrome. *Br. Med. J.*, **297**, 1024–6
5. Adashi, E.J., Rock, J.A., Guzick, D., Wentz, A.C., Jones, G.S. and Jones, H.W. Jr. (1981). Fertility following bilateral ovarian wedge resection: a critical analysis of 90 consecutive cases of the polycystic ovary syndrome. *Fertil. Steril.*, **36**, 320–5
6. Garcea, N., Campo, S., Panetta, V., Venneri, M., Siccardi, P., Dargenio, R. and De Tomasi, F. (1985). Induction of ovulation with purified urinary follicle stimulating hormone in patients with polycystic ovarian syndrome. *Am. J. Obstet. Gynecol.*, **151**, 635–40
7. Rönnberg, L., Ylöstalo, P. and Ruokonen, A. (1985). Hormonal parameters and conception rate during five different types of treatment of polycystic ovarian syndrome. *Int. J. Gynaecol. Obstet.*, **23**, 177–83
8. Sagle, M., Bishop, K., Ridley, N., Alexander, F.M., Michel, M., Bonney, R.C., Beard, R.W. and Franks, S. (1988). Recurrent early miscarriage and polycystic ovaries. *Br. Med. J.*, **297**, 1027–8
9. Plachot, M., de Grouchy, J., Junca, A.M., Mandelbaum, J., Salat-Baroux, J. and Cohen, J. (1988). Chromosome analysis of human oocytes and embryos: does delayed fertilization increase chromosome imbalance? *Hum. Reprod.*, **3**, 125–7
10. Homburg, R. and Jacobs, H.S. (1989). Etiology of miscarriage in polycystic ovary syndrome. *Fertil. Steril.*, **51**, 196
11. Seibel, M.M., Smith, D., Dlugli, A.M. and Levesque, L. (1989). Periovulatory follicular fluid hormone levels in spontaneous human cycles. *J. Clin. Endocrinol. Metab.*, **68**, 1073–7
12. Lobo, R.A., DiZerega, A. and Marrs, R.P. (1985). Follicular fluid steroid levels in dysmature and mature follicles from spontaneous and hyperstimulated cycles in normal and anovulatory women. *J. Clin. Endocrinol. Metab.*, **60**, 81–7
13. Hammond, M.G., Halme, J. and Talbert, L.M. (1985). Gamete quality and fertility regulation. In Rolland, R. *et al.* (eds.) *Pelvic Macrophages as Modulators of Human Granulosa Cell Progesterone Production*, pp. 73–81. (Amsterdam: Elsevier Science)
14. Scialli, A.R. (1986). The reproductive toxicity of ovulation induction. *Fertil. Steril.*, **45**, 315–23
15. Garcia, J., Jones, G.S. and Wentz, A.C. (1977). The use of clomiphene citrate. *Fertil. Steril.*, **28**, 707–17
16. Plachot, M., de Grouchy, J. and Salat-Baroux, J. (1989). Genetics of human oocytes. Presented at *The XIIth World Congress on Fertility and Sterility*. Marrakesh, Abstr. p. 609
17. Testart, J., Belaisch-Allart, J., Forman, R., Gazengel, A., Strubb, N., Hazout, A. and Frydman, R. (1989). Influence of different stimulation treatments on oocyte characteristics and *in-vitro* fertilizing ability. *Hum. Reprod.*, **4**, 192–7
18. Testart, J., Forman, R., Belaisch-Allart, J., Volante, M., Hazout, A., Strubb, N. and Frydman, R. (1989). Embryo quality and uterine receptivity in *in-vitro* fertilization cycles with or without agonists of gonadotropin-releasing hormone. *Hum. Reprod.*, **4**, 198–201
19. Bilowus, M., Abbassi, V. and Gibbons, M.D. (1986). Female pseudohermaphroditism in a neonate born to a mother with polycystic ovarian disease. *J. Urol.*, **136**, 1098–100
20. Berger, N.C., Repke, J.T. and Woodruff, J.D. (1984). Markedly elevated serum testosterone in pregnancy without fetal virilization. *Am. J. Obstet. Gynecol.*, **63**, 260–2
21. Thompson, C.R. and Hansen, L.A. (1970). Pergonal (Menotropins): a summary of clinical experience in the induction of ovulation and pregnancy. *Fertil. Steril.*, **21**, 844–53
22. Wang, C.F. and Gemzell, C. (1980). The use of human gonadotropins for the induction of ovulation in women with polycystic ovarian disease. *Fertil. Steril.*, **33**, 479–86
23. Fleming, R., Jamieson, M.P.R., Hamilton, M.P.R., Black, W.P., MacNaughton, M.C. and

Coutts, J.R.T. (1988). The use of GnRH analogues in combination with exogenous gonadotropins in infertile women. *Acta Endocrinol.*, **288**, 77–84

24. Remorgida, V., Venturini, P.L., Anserini, P., Lanera, P. and De Cecco, L. (1989). Administration of pure follicle-stimulation hormone during gonadotropin releasing hormone agonist therapy in patients with clomiphene-resistant polycystic ovarian disease: hormonal evaluations and clinical perspectives. *Am. J. Obstet. Gynecol.*, **160**, 108–13

25. Burger, C.W., Korsen, T.J.M., Hompes, P.G.A., van Kessel, H. and Schoemaker, J. (1986). Ovulation induction with pulsatile luteinizing releasing hormone in women with clomiphene citrate-resistant polycystic ovary-like disease: clinical results. *Fertil. Steril.*, **46**, 1045–54

26. Ashkenazi, J., Feldberg, D., Dicker, D., Yeshaya, A., Ayalon, D. and Goldman, J.A. (1989). IVF-ET in women with refractory polycystic ovarian disease. *Eur. J. Obstet. Gynecol. Reprod. Biol.*, **30**, 157–61

27. Gjönaess, H. (1989). The course and outcome of pregnancy after ovarian electrocautery in women with polycystic ovarian syndrome: the influence of body-weight. *Br. J. Obstet. Gynaecol.*, **96**, 714–19

20

Long-term management of patients with chronic hyperandrogenic anovulation

J.V.T.H. Hamerlynck

INTRODUCTION

From previous chapters it is clear that, apart from infertility, patients with chronic hyperandrogenic anovulation (CHA) or polycystic ovary syndrome (PCOS) may present with several different complaints or problems such as amenorrhea or dysfunctional uterine bleedings, hirsutism and even virilism, and obesity. It is also clear that some patients, even without definite complaints, are at risk in several respects. At first there is the association of increased insulin resistance and, consequently, disturbance of glucose homeostasis[1]. Furthermore, there is a definitely increased risk of developing endometrial hyperplasia and endometrial carcinoma. Also continuous unopposed hyperestrogenism may lead to a higher prevalence of breast disease[2]. Finally, the unfavorable lipoprotein profile puts them at risk of cardiovascular disease[3]. So, for many reasons, patients with CHA without any doubt need to be followed and to be treated not only for occasional complaints, but also, and this is even more important, in order to prevent risks in the long term.

HYPERANDROGENISM AND HYPERESTROGENISM

Apart from hyperandrogenism, unopposed hyperestrogenism is the other pathogenetic key for many of the problems and risks in CHA. As we know, not only hyperandrogenism but also hyperestrogenism contribute to the state of persistent anovulation (70%) and amenorrhea (55%).

Hyperandrogenism may, in addition, be chiefly responsible for hirsutism and virilism as well as for an increased appetite and obesity and, finally, for an unfavorable lipoprotein profile and cardiovascular risk[3].

Hyperestrogenism is considered to be responsible for irregular, sometimes heavy, bleedings (30%) and for a three- to fourfold increased risk of the development of endometrial carcinoma and an equally increased risk of breast cancer[2].

Finally, the well-recognized correlation between increased insulin resistance and chronic hyperandrogenic anovulation, regardless of body weight or the presence of obesity, is another aspect which deserves special attention[1].

PRECAUTIONS BEFORE STARTING TREATMENT

Diagnosis of CHA is easily made and is discussed elsewhere. The typical patient presents with amenorrhea (or irregular menses with periods of amenorrhea) and has a withdrawal bleeding after a progestogen challenge test.

Even in the absence of hirsutism, an endometrial biopsy and a mammography are wise precautions in any patient who has long-standing anovulation before starting therapy. An oral glucose tolerance test is also essential.

LONG-TERM PREVENTATIVE AND THERAPEUTIC MANAGEMENT OF CHA (PCO) PATIENTS

Treatment with progestogens

The obvious treatment of an anovulatory patient with complaints of amenorrhea or dysfunctional bleedings, presenting with a positive progestogen challenge test or with other signs of hyperestrogenic activity such as abundant liquid cervical mucus, is the administration of progesterone or progestogens. Dysfunctional bleedings will cease and regular withdrawal bleedings will appear.

If administered in adequate dosages and during an adequate number of days per cycle or per month, endometrial hyperplasia will not develop and, if present, it will (probably) be adequately treated, thereby reducing the risk of developing endometrial carcinoma in the long term even below the overall risk in the normal population[4].

Possibly, the same applies for the risk of developing breast disease although adequate follow-up studies in this respect are still missing[5]. On the other hand, treatment with progestogens will have no influence at all on the early and late unfavorable effects of hyperandrogenism, since the treatment has no significant effect on production of androgen by the ovaries. Administration of progestogens should therefore be restricted as a therapy for anovulatory patients, either without pronounced hyperandrogenism, or with either objections to or side-effects from other therapies. Finally, it should be mentioned that long-term administration of progestogens highlights the importance of the right choice of progestagenic compounds. As a general rule, C-21 compounds (progesterone itself, dydrogesterone, medroxyprogesterone acetate, megestrol acetate) should be preferred over nortestosterone derivatives, as all of the latter have some androgenic effects which are generally absent or less pronounced in C-21 compounds[6].

In order to prevent endometrial hyperplasia, additive progestogen therapy is essential for at least 10 days and preferably 12 days per month and the necessary dose for each progestogen (based on adequate transformation of proliferative endometrium into secretory endometrium) is now well documented[7].

Treatment with antiandrogens

The most potent antiandrogen is probably cyproterone acetate, a C-21 progestogen compound with a strong blocking action on androgen receptors, for example in the hair follicles. It also has inhibitory effects on ovarian steroidogenesis, particularly in high doses[8]. It is a generally well-tolerated potent progestational agent and is often prescribed in doses of 100 mg daily in combination (in a reversed sequential regime as proposed by Hammerstein) with 50 μg ethinylestradiol[9]. This scheme has a pronounced negative feedback effect on luteinizing hormone releasing hormone (LHRH) and gonadotropin release, which also means that ovarian steroidogenesis becomes depressed. The combination with high doses of ethinylestradiol has the advantage that levels of circulating sex hormone binding globulin (SHBG) increase, which leads to more binding of testosterone and an important lowering of free (active) testosterone. Some occasional side-effects such as loss of libido, weight gain, headache and mastalgia deserve attention and may necessitate lowering of the dose (in particular the dose of ethinylestradiol). Hirsutism (facial) especially improves usually significantly after 3–6 months of treatment. As this treatment has a depressive effect on ovarian steroidogenesis and androgen production with consequent regulation of menses and improvement of the lipoprotein profile, it may be the long-term treatment of choice for chronic hyperandrogenic anovulatory patients. Incidentally, however, a marked depression of libido occurs and together with some other already mentioned side-effects, which in fact are probably more estrogenic in origin, this means that the Hammerstein scheme should be reserved for seriously androgenized (hirsute) women only.

Another potential drawback is that the treatment may exacerbate hyperinsulinemia with concomitant deterioration of glucose tolerance in PCO patients with a history of gestational diabetes[10].

Sometimes a lowering of dose of both cyproterone acetate and ethinylestradiol may lead to adequate effects and acceptance in the long term. However, one must ensure that contraception remains guaranteed, since 'escape' ovulations may result in conceptions and feminization of the male fetus.

The same goes for other antiandrogens such as spironolactone, which also has a competing effect on the androgen receptor and an inhibitory effect on ovarian as well as on adrenal androgen production[11]. It seems wise to prescribe spironolactone in combination with a birth control pill, which, as we shall see, in itself has a favorable effect on ovarian androgen production. Spironolactone, in combination with oral contraceptives, is an efficacious and well-tolerated approach to the management of hirsutism which is unresponsive to oral contraceptives alone.

Dexamethasone depresses only adrenal androgen secretion and is therefore not suitable as a mode of treatment for chronic patients with CHA.

Oral contraceptive agents

Since it has been shown *in vitro* that the hyperplastic thecal cells are a significant site of abnormal androgen production and appear more sensitive to human chorionic gonadotropin (hCG) than thecal cells from normal ovaries[12], it seems logical that artificial depression of the LH impulse results in a depression of ovarian androgen production. In this respect the studies of Cullberg and colleagues[13,14] are relevant. Using a contraceptive agent containing 0.150 mg desogestrel and 0.030 mg ethinylestradiol, a suppression of increased total and free testosterone levels was evident; moreover, an increase of SHBG capacity became apparent.

In addition, in an ultrasound study Venturoli showed that contraceptive therapy temporarily restored normal ovarian morphology in subjects with polycystic ovaries[15]. Most of the patients in a study by Rojanasakul and colleagues showed an improvement of androgenic symptoms[16]. However, long-term treatment may be needed since the abnormal menstrual pattern reappeared soon after cessation of pill intake.

The ratio of low-density lipoprotein cholesterol to high-density lipoprotein cholesterol, although showing no significant change, had a tendency to decrease[17].

Therefore, the use of contraceptive agents is a very valuable mode of long-term treatment of preferably young patients with mild to moderate CHA: bleedings are regulated, endometrial hyperplasia will not occur and ovarian androgen effects such as hirsutism will not develop or increase. The lipoprotein profile will also probably be influenced favorably. Self-evidently, the patient remains protected from unwanted fertility (escape ovulations).

The surgical option

Bilateral ovarian wedge resection (BOWR) in patients with polycystic ovary syndrome resistant to clomiphene (combined with hCG) is considered nowadays to be a rather obsolete procedure. The main reason is the widespread and relatively successful use of gonadotropins (human menopausal gonadotropin and pure follicle stimulating hormone) for induction of ovulation in PCO patients under adequate ultrasound monitoring. Another reason is that generally regular menses can develop after BOWR, but only in a relatively small number of patients does the restoration of ovulatory cycles (with normalization of endocrine parameters, including the ultrasound aspect of the ovaries) lead to conceptions and pregnancies. This is mainly due to filmy adhesions enveloping the operated ovaries which interfere with a normal tubo-ovarian interaction, as has been shown at second-look laparoscopy in 90% of the treated patients[18].

BOWR by electrocautery[19] or by laser vaporization[20] or other technical procedures has produced fewer adhesions and a higher conception rate but often, after a while, recurrence of the PCO syndrome has developed. So the threat of an early recurrence of PCO (sometimes after only a few months) is another drawback of BOWR. It has been suggested that the main reason for recurrence consists in the relatively small number of androgen-producing cells that are removed by BOWR or alternative surgical procedures. Massive removal of androgen-producing cells by unilateral ovariectomy seems to result in a long-term restoration of ovulatory cyclicity in the remaining ovary in rats with experimentally induced PCO[21] as well as in women[22]. In six unilaterally ovariectomized PCOS patients who could be followed for at least 10 years, except for some temporary periods of anovulation, no recurrence of the disease could be detected. After surgery, immediate normalization of the endocrine parameters and normal ovulatory cyclicity appeared and persisted, a highly satisfactory outcome for the patients. Sometimes hirsutism still had to be treated with antiandrogens, but after cessation of therapy reappearance of hair growth was very mild and certainly not excessive (Hamerlynck, J. and Chan, E., unpublished).

There can be no doubt that for CHA (PCO) patients wishing to have a child, the surgical procedures to achieve this goal are considered to be an obsolete option in view of the vast progress that has been made in methods of ovulation induction and in the improvement in monitoring follicle growth and ovulation using endocrine parameters and ultrasound. In the management of patients who do not wish to have a child, however, the surgical approach in our view remains a valid option, at least if a long-term restoration of ovulatory cyclicity can be obtained and confirmed (unilateral ovariectomy). This small intervention can possibly lead to a complete recovery from the syndrome, eliminating cycle disturbances and the increased risks of endometrial hyperplasia and carcinoma. It also eliminates unfavorable lipoprotein profiles and the increased risk of vascular problems in the long term. If necessary, complaints such as hirsutism and android obesity are more easily treated by conventional methods.

The benefit of the surgical therapeutical option still has to be confirmed in a large number of patients not wishing to have a child, preferably patients with large polycystic ovaries and suffering seriously from the known PCO problems.

CONCLUSION

Women with chronic hyperandrogenic anovulation and/or polycystic ovary syndrome deserve continuing attention, in view of their complaints, problems or risks in the long term, even after having had a child. Long-term management and treatment of these patients may be of great importance. In mildly to moderately affected women, oral contraceptive agents appear to be preferred over the simple administration of progestogens only. In more seriously affected and androgenized patients, antiandrogens, preferably incorporated in a scheme with estrogens, seem to be the treatment of choice, although a surgical approach cannot be considered as an obsolete option.

REFERENCES

1. Smith, S., Ravnikar, Y.A. and Barbieri, R.L. (1987). Androgen and insulin response to an oral glucose challenge in hyperandrogenic women. *Fertil. Steril.*, **48**, 72

2. Coulam, C.B., Annegers, J.F. and Kranz, J.S. (1983). Chronic anovulation syndrome and associated neoplasia. *Obstet. Gynecol.*, **61**, 403
3. Wild, R.A., Painter, P.C., Coulson, P.B., Carruth, K.B. and Ranney, G.B. (1985). Lipoprotein lipid concentrations and cardiovascular risk in women with polycystic ovary syndrome. *J. Clin. Endocrinol. Metab.*, **61**, 46
4. Gambrell, R.D. Jr., Babgnell, C.A. and Greenblatt, R.B. (1983). Role of estrogens and progesterone in the etiology and prevention of endometrial cancer: a review. *Am. J. Obstet. Gynecol.*, **146**, 696
5. Gambrell, R.D. Jr., Maier, R. and Sangers, B.I. (1983). Decreased incidence of breast cancer in postmenopausal estrogen–progestogen users. *Obstet. Gynecol.*, **62**, 435
6. Lobo, R.A. (1987). Absorption and metabolic effects of different types of estrogens and progestogens. *Obstet. Gynecol. Clin. N. Am.*, **14**, 143
7. Whitehead, M.I. and Fraser, D. (1987). The effects of estrogens and progestogens on the endometrium. *Obstet. Gynecol. Clin. N. Am.*, **14**, 299
8. Holdeway, I.M., Croxson, M.S., Ibbertson, H.R., Sheeman, A., Knox, B. and France, J. (1985). Cyproterone acetate as initial treatment and maintenance therapy for hirsutism. *Acta Endocrinol.*, **109**, 522
9. Venturoli, S., Paradisi, R., Saviotti, E., Porcu, E., Fabbri, R., Orsini, L.F., Bovicelli, L. and Flamigni, C. (1985). Ultrasound study of ovarian and uterine morphology in women with polycystic ovary syndrome before, during and after treatment with cyproterone acetate and ethinylestradiol. *Arch. Gynecol.*, **237**, 1
10. Plehwe, W.E., Maitland, J.E., Williams, P.F., Shearman, R.P. and Turtie, J.R. (1985). Familial hyperinsulinemia complicated by extreme insulin resistance during pregnancy: a probable postreceptor defect. *J. Clin. Endocrinol. Metab.*, **61**, 68
11. Milewicz, A., Silber, D. and Kirschner, M.A. (1983). Therapeutic effects of spironolactone in polycystic ovary syndrome. *Obstet. Gynecol.*, **61**, 429
12. Dennefors, B.L., Knutson, F., Janson, P.O., Jansson, I. and Hamberger, L. (1985). Ovarian steroid production in a woman with polycystic ovary syndrome associated with endometrial cancer. *Acta Obstet. Gynecol. Scand.*, **64**, 387
13. Cullberg, G. (1985). Pharmacodynamic studies on desogestrel administered alone and in combination with ethinylestradiol. *Acta Obstet. Gynecol. Scand.*, Suppl. **133**, 1
14. Cullberg, G., Hamberger, L., Mattson, L.A., Mobacken, H. and Samsioe, G. (1985). Effects of a low-dose desogestrel–ethinylestradiol combination on hirsutism, androgens and sex hormone binding globulin in women with a polycystic ovary syndrome. *Acta Obstet. Gynecol. Scand.*, **64**, 195
15. Venturoli, S., Paradisi, R., Saviotti, E., Barnabe, S., Porcu, E., Fabbri, R. and Flamigni, C. (1983). Ultrasound study of ovarian morphology in women with polycystic ovary syndrome before and during treatment with an oestrogen/progestagen preparation. *Arch. Gynecol.*, **234**, 87
16. Rojanasakul, A., Sirimongkolkasem, R., Priomsawasdi, S., Sumavong, V., Chailurkit, L. and Chaturachinda, K. (1987). Effects of combined ethinylestradiol and desogestrel on hormone profiles and sex hormone binding globulin in women with polycystic ovarian disease. *Contraception*, **36**, 633
17. Rojanasakul, A., Chailurkit, L., Sirimongkolkasem, R. and Chaturachinda, K. (1987). Effects of combined desogestrel–ethinylestradiol treatment on lipid profiles in women with polycystic ovarian disease. *Fertil. Steril.*, **48**, 581
18. Portuondo, J.A., Melchor, J.C., Neyre, J.L. and Alegre, A. (1984). Periovarian adhesions following ovarian wedge resection or laparoscopic biopsy. *Endoscopy*, **16**, 143
19. Greenblatt, E. and Casper, R.F. (1987). Endocrine changes after laparoscopic ovarian cautery in polycystic ovarian syndrome. *Am. J. Obstet. Gynecol.*, **156**, 279
20. Daniell, J.F. and Miller, W. (1989). Polycystic ovaries treated by laparoscopic laser vaporization. *Fertil. Steril.*, **51**, 232
21. Farookhi, R., Hemmings, R. and Brawer, J.R. (1985). Unilateral ovariectomy restores ovarian cyclicity in rats with a polycystic ovarian condition. *Biol. Reprod.*, **32**, 530
22. Hamerlynck, J.V.T.H. (1982). Polycystic ovaries disease: one ovary too many? *Lancet*, **2**, 937

21

Chronic anovulation and endometrial carcinoma

F.M. Helmerhorst and T.J.M. Helmerhorst

HISTORY

The story of chronic anovulation and endometrial carcinoma started in 1935 (Table 1). In that year Stein and Leventhal described a syndrome characterized by secondary amenorrhea, anovulation, infertility and bilateral enlarged ovaries. Many of the affected patients were hirsute and obese.

In that same year of 1935, Robinson[2] remarked on the association of enlarged polycystic ovaries with metrorrhagia due to cystic hyperplasia of the endometrium. In 1948, Woll and his associates[3] described the features of cortical stromal hyperplasia of the ovaries, which they found to be approximately twice as common in live women with carcinoma of the endometrium as in women of similar age without carcinoma, whose ovaries were examined at autopsy. In 1949 Speert associated corpus malignancy with polycystic ovary syndrome in young women[4]. Other authors such as Novak and Mohler[5] and Schneider and Bechtel[7] subsequently confirmed the findings of these investigators and suggested that the hyperplastic ovarian stroma, by secreting estrogens, had a role in the development of endometrial

Table 1 History of polycystic ovary syndrome (PCOS) and endometrial carcinoma

Year	Author	Discovery
1935	Stein and Leventhal[1]	the syndrome
	Robinson[2]	association between polycystic ovaries and endometrial hyperplasia
1948	Woll et al.[3]	association between polycystic ovaries and endometrial carcinoma
1949	Speert[4]	association between polycystic ovaries and endometrial carcinoma in young women
1953	Novak and Mohler[5]	estrogens involved in the development of corpus cancer in PCOS patients
1975	Dallenbach-Hellweg[6]	atypical endometrial hyperplasia as a premalignant condition for endometrial carcinoma

carcinoma. Morphological criteria of the different types of endometrial hyperplasia (including atypical hyperplasia) as a premalignant condition were first described by Dallenbach-Hellweg[6].

EPIDEMIOLOGY

The general risk of endometrial carcinoma is estimated as 1 per 1000 untreated postmenopausal women per year[8]. During the last decades the incidence of endometrial carcinoma has not been a constant figure. Quint was the first in 1975 to report on the changing and increased incidence of endometrial adenocarcinoma[9]. In that year two studies were published in the same issue of *The New England Journal of Medicine* suggesting the relationship between the increased risk of developing endometrial adenocarcinoma and the administration of exogenous estrogens[10,11]. The estrogens were administered to very considerable numbers of women, largely as postmenopausal hormone replacement therapy. Of the women suffering from adenocarcinoma, 95% were older than 40 years. The corpus cancer of these patients was predominantly related with exogenous estrogens. However, in studies on endometrial cancer in patients *under* 40 years old, obesity and chronic anovulation were the predominant factors[12,13].

Gallup and Stock[14], as well as Fahri and colleagues[15], found endometrial adenocarcinoma in young women with polycystic ovary syndrome, as shown on Table 2.

In 1957 Jackson and Dockerty[16] reported a 27% frequency of development of endometrial carcinoma in women with polycystic ovaries of the type described by Stein and Leventhal[1]. Coulan[17] reported in 1983 that the risk of adenocarcinoma of the endometrium was increased by long-term chronic anovulation. The relative risk was calculated as 5.

The relationship between hyperplasia of the endometrium and endometrial carcinoma will be discussed later in this paper. It is important here to notice the risk of endometrial adenocarcinoma in women with a diagnosed endometrial hyperplasia. In a group of 24 young women with endometrial hyperplasia studied by Chamlian and Taylor in 1970, followed up to 14 years, three patients (12.5%) developed endometrial carcinoma[18]. Other investigators found 18 and 50% after a period of time[19,20].

PATHOPHYSIOLOGY

The association between estrogen and uterine cancer may have first been made by Schröder in 1922 when he reported an individual developing

Table 2 Polycystic ovary syndrome (PCOS) in patients with endometrial adenocarcinoma

	Number of patients with PCOS		
	15–25 years	*29–40 years*	*> 40 years*
Gallup and Stock[14]		5/16	2/95
Fahri *et al.*[15]	7/10		

endometrial adenocarcinoma in conjunction with a estrogen-secreting granulosa cell tumor of the ovary[21]. Additional support for estrogen being a contributing factor in the development of hyperplasia and endometrial carcinoma is derived indirectly from the association of uterine adenocarcinoma with chronic hyperestrogenic states such as estrogen-secreting ovarian tumors[22,23] and hepatocellular disease[24] resulting in impaired estrogen metabolism. Direct evidence that estrogens are a potential endometrial carcinogen was obtained from observations in women with non-functioning gonads who used exogenous estrogens. In these patients treated for 4–20 years with estrogens, adenocarcinoma of the endometrium has developed at 40 years or younger, whereas in those with gonadal dysgenesis not treated with estrogen, endometrial cancer has not developed with only one exception, according to Cutler and colleagues[25].

What is the mode of action of estrogens in the development of endometrial adenocarcinoma? Before the estrogen can cause growth of the endometrium, it has to react with a receptor protein in the endometrial cell. The estrogen is transported into the nucleus and is retained within the nucleus for a sufficient period of time to initiate DNA synthesis and cell proliferation. Estradiol seems a considerably more potent steroid than estrone in binding to the nucleus of the endometrial cells. In this model, estrogens have proliferative effects on the endometrium; however, evidence of a direct mutagenic effect is lacking.

In theory, steroids can induce neoplasia by a number of different mechanisms, such as:

(1) Direct carcinogenic effect;

(2) Stimulation or production of other hormones with carcinogenic effects;

(3) Synergistic action to stimulate proliferation in tissues subjected to environmental carcinogens;

(4) Transformation of chemical agents into carcinogens by metabolic changes;

(5) Modification of the immune response.

The use of exogenous estrogens suggested a causative role of this steroid in developing endometrial cancer. The risk of endometrial cancer being positively correlated with duration of exposure and dosage led to the hypothesis of unopposed estrogen action (by progestogens)[19]. This hypothesis implies that estrogens generate atypical cells by enhancing cell proliferation and by additional effects.

Fox pointed out that 'there is little to indicate that oestrogens act as an initiator rather than as a promoter of endometrial adenocarcinoma. It is suggested that oestrogens promote cell proliferation of cells in which a malignant change has been previously initiated'[26].

Table 3 shows a compilation of studies on the detection of estrone and estradiol in the peripheral blood and the ovarian veins in patients with polycystic ovary syndrome. The conclusion can be drawn from the data presented that the estrogen level is constantly increased in patients with polycystic ovary syndrome.

Table 3 Estrogen levels in PCOS patients

Reference		Estrone	Estradiol
Baird et al.[27]		↑	↑
DeVane et al.[28]		↑	as in early follicular phase
Judd[29]		↑	as in early follicular phase
Lobo et al.[30]		↑	total and unbound ↑
Laatikainen et al.[31]			ovarian vein: normal range
Kasuga[32]	ovarian vein	↑	↑
	peripheral	↓	↑

Since women with polycystic ovary syndrome produce three to four times more androstenedione than normal[33], one can raise the question whether androgens play a role in the development of endometrial cancer. However, although the incidence of androgen-secreting ovarian tumors is low, no remarkable changes in the endometrium have been found[34].

Is hyperplasia of the endometrium an intermediate state towards corpus carcinoma? The association between a previously diagnosed hyperplasia and carcinoma of the endometrium has already been described by Cullen in 1900[35]. In 1974 Wentz reported the fate of 115 patients with adenomatous hyperplasia or adenocarcinoma *in situ* of the endometrium[20] (Table 4).

The patients were withheld from hormonal or surgical therapy. Nearly 50% of the patients developed an invasive adenocarcinoma of the endometrium within a period of 2–8 years. From this and other studies[36], we may conclude that hyperplasia of the endometrium is a precancerous lesion and can progress to endometrial carcinoma.

PROGNOSIS

There is general consensus that adenocarcinomas of the endometrium developing in hyperestrogenized patients are usually at an early stage, well differentiated, and tend to invade only to the inner third of the myometrium. In these patients the 5-year survival rate is 92%. The 5-year rate for women with non-estrogen-related endometrial neoplasms is 67%[26]. Robboy and Bradley[37] described a frequency of 12% poorly differentiated adenocarcinoma in estrogen users, as compared with 37% in non-users. In the literature[38], three cases with endometrial sarcoma complicating PCOS have been reported. In conclusion, corpus cancer in polycystic ovary syndrome patients is a relatively benign malignancy.

Table 4 From hyperplasia to carcinoma[20]

Pathology	Number of patients	% developing adenocarcinoma
Adenomatous hyperplasia	75	26.7
Atypical hyperplasia	22	81.0
Adenocarcinoma *in situ*	18	100.0
Total	115	48.7

PREVENTION

When progestogens are cyclically given with estrogen to menopausal women, a decrease in the incidence of endometrial cancer has been observed[39]. The efficacy of the progestogen therapy has been demonstrated[40-42]. Progestogens inhibit the synthesis of these estrogen receptors and thus, when given with an estrogen, prevent the growth-promoting action of the estrogen. Another mechanism of the progestogen protection against endometrial cancer induced by estrogens is the elimination of the endometrial cells and glands by shedding[43].

Studd and colleagues[41] and Whitehead and colleagues[42] recommend the minimal duration of cyclic progestogens of 13 days each month (see also ref. 44), in postmenopausal estrogen replacement therapy. However, some focal areas of the endometrium and rarely the full endometrium do not seem to respond to progestogen: an 100% protection by the progestogen therapy cannot be achieved[45]. Progestogens administered during 13 days per month to patients with proven benign hyperplasia are 98% effective in changing the hyperplasia to normal endometrium[13,46]. A curettage after 3 and 6 months should be repeated to ensure that all hyperplasia has been distinguished and eradicated[43]. Gambrell[43] recommends hysterectomy when the atypical hyperplasia progresses after 3 months or is still present after 6 months. When in this case infertility is also involved, it is sometimes very difficult to decide for hysterectomy. Muechler[47] described the following case in *Fertility and Sterility* in 1986: 'A 31-year-old woman is described with PCOD associated with endometrial hyperplasia and well-differentiated adenocarcinoma. Conservative treatment with ovulation induction was pursued for a total of $3\frac{1}{2}$ years. After clomiphene citrate treatment failed to achieve conception, treatment with menotropins resulted in a twin pregnancy that aborted spontaneously and a singleton term pregnancy. Hysterectomy was performed $4\frac{1}{2}$ years after the initial diagnosis of well-differentiated endometrial adenocarcinoma was made. Histological examination of the endometrium showed no progression of the disease. Ovulation induction of patients with polycystic ovaries and well-differentiated and non-invasive endometrial adenocarcinoma may be justified in properly selected cases.'

PCOS patients without the wish to conceive are advised to use a low-dose estrogen–progestogen combination contraceptive pill, since there is substantial evidence of a decrease in frequency of endometrial adenocarcinoma in those patients compared with non-pill users[48-51].

CLOSING REMARKS

Polycystic ovary syndrome in a hyperestrogenized condition is a substantial risk in the development of endometrial adenocarcinoma. Atypical hyperplasia can be detected with an endometrial biopsy or a curettage. One can prevent the endometrial hyperplasia and carcinoma in these patients by a 13-day progestogen treatment inducing a monthly shedding of the endometrium.

REFERENCES

1. Stein, I.F. and Leventhal, M.L. (1935). Amenorrhea associated with bilateral polycystic ovaries. *Am. J. Obstet. Gynecol.*, **29**, 181–91
2. Robinson, M.R. (1935). The surgical treatment of ovarian dysfunctions. *Am. J. Obstet. Gynecol.*, **30**, 18–36
3. Woll, E., Hertig, A.T., Smith, G.V.S. and Johnson, L.C. (1948). The ovary in endometrial carcinoma. *Am. J. Obstet. Gynecol.*, **56**, 617–33
4. Speert, H. (1949). Cancer of the endometrium in young women. *Surg. Gynecol. Obstet.*, **88**, 332–6
5. Novak, E.R. and Mohler, D.I. (1953). Ovarian stromal changes in endometrial cancer. *Am. J. Obstet. Gynecol.*, **65**, 1099–110
6. Dallenbach-Hellweg, G. (1975). In *Histopathology of the Endometrium*. (Berlin, New York: Springer Verlag)
7. Schneider, G.T. and Bechtel, M. (1956). Ovarian cortical stromal hyperplasia. *Obstet. Gynecol.*, **8**, 713–19
8. Weiss, N.S. (1975). Risks and benefits of estrogen use. *N. Engl. J. Med.*, **293**, 1200–2
9. Quint, B.C. (1975). Changing patterns in endometrial adenocarcinoma. *Am. J. Obstet. Gynecol.*, **122**, 498–501
10. Smith, D.C., Prentice, R., Thompson, D.J. and Herrmann, W.L. (1975). Association of exogenous estrogen and endometrial carcinoma. *N. Engl. J. Med.*, **293**, 1164–7
11. Ziel, H.K. and Finkle, W.D. (1975). Increased risk of endometrial carcinoma among users of conjugated estrogens. *N. Engl. J. Med.*, **293**, 1167–70
12. Peterson, E.P. (1968). Endometrial carcinoma in young women: a clinical profile. *Obstet. Gynecol.*, **31**, 702–7
13. Fechner, R.E. and Kaufman, R.H. (1974). Endometrial adenocarcinoma in Stein–Leventhal syndrome. *Cancer*, **34**, 444–52
14. Gallup, D.G. and Stock, R.J. (1984). Adenocarcinoma of the endometrium in women 40 years of age or younger. *Obstet. Gynecol.*, **64**, 417–20
15. Fahri, D.C., Nosanchuk, J. and Silverberg, S.G. (1986). Endometrial adenocarcinoma in women under 25 years of age. *Obstet. Gynecol.*, **68**, 741–5
16. Jackson, R.L. and Dockerty, M.B. (1957). The Stein–Leventhal syndrome: analysis of 43 cases with special reference to association with endometrial carcinoma. *Am. J. Obstet. Gynecol.*, **73**, 161–73
17. Coulan, C.B., Annegers, J.F. and Kranz, J.S. (1983). Chronic anovulation syndrome and associated neoplasia. *Obstet. Gynecol.*, **61**, 403–7
18. Chamlian, D.L. and Taylor, H.B. (1970). Endometrial hyperplasia in young women. *Obstet. Gynecol.*, **36**, 659–66
19. Gusberg, S.B. (1976). The individual at high-risk for endometrial carcinoma. *Am. J. Obstet. Gynecol.*, **126**, 535–42
20. Wentz, W.B. (1974). Progestin therapy in endometrial hyperplasia. *Gynecol. Oncol.*, **2**, 362–7
21. Schröder, R. (1922). Granulosazelltumor des Ovars mit glandulärcystischer Hyperplasie des Endometriums und beginnendem Karzinom auf diesem Boden. *Zentralbl. Gynäkol.*, **46**, 195–6
22. Ingram, J.M. and Novak, E. (1951). Endometrial carcinoma associated with feminizing ovarian tumors. *Am. J. Obstet. Gynecol.*, **61**, 774–87
23. Greene, J.W. (1957). Feminizing mesenchymomas (granulosa and theca cell tumors) with associated endometrial carcinoma: review of the literature and a study of the material of the Ovarian Tumor Registry. *Am. J. Obstet. Gynecol.*, **74**, 31–41
24. MacDonald, P.C. and Siiteri, P.K. (1974). The relationship between the extraglandular production of estrone and the occurrence of endometrial neopolasia. *Gynecol. Oncol.*, **2**, 259–63
25. Cutler, B.S., Forbes, A.P., Ingersoll, F.M. and Scully, R.E. (1972). Endometrial carcinoma after stilbestrol therapy in gonadal dysgenesis. *N. Engl. J. Med.*, **287**, 628–31
26. Fox, H. (1984). Endometrial carcinogenesis and its relation to oestrogens. *Path. Res. Pract.*, **179**, 13–19

27. Baird, D.T., Corker, C.S., Davidson, D.W., Hunter, W.M., Michie, E.A. and Look, P.F.A. van (1977). Pituitary–ovarian relationships in polycystic ovary syndrome. *J. Clin. Endocrinol. Metab.*, **45**, 798–809

28. DeVane, G.W., Czekala, N.M., Judd, H.L. and Yen, S.S.C. (1975). Circulating gonadotropins, estrogens, and androgens in polycystic ovarian disease. *Am. J. Obstet. Gynecol.*, **121**, 496–500

29. Judd, H.L. (1978). Endocrinology of polycystic ovarian disease. *Clin. Obstet. Gynecol.*, **21**, 99–114

30. Lobo, R.A., Granger, L., Goebelsmann, U. and Mishell, D.R. (1981). Elevations in unbound serum estradiol as a possible mechanism for inappropriate gonadotropin secretion in women with PCO. *J. Clin. Endocrinol. Metab.*, **52**, 156–8

31. Laatikainen, T.J., Apter, D.L., Paavonen, J.A. and Wahlström, T.R. (1980). Steroids in ovarian and peripheral venous blood in polycystic ovarian disease. *Clin. Endocrinol.*, **13**, 125–34

32. Kasuga, Y. (1980). Ovarian steroidogenesis in Japanese patients with polycystic ovary syndrome. *Endocrinol. Jpn.*, **27**, 541–50

33. Siiteri, P.K. and MacDonald, P.C. (1973). Role of extraglandular estrogen in human endocrinology. In Geiger, S.R., Astwood, E.B. and Greep, R.O. (eds.) *Handbook of Physiology*, pp. 615–29. (The American Physiology Society)

34. Kühnel, R. (1986). Steroid hormone receptors in human ovarian cancer. *Thesis*, Amsterdam

35. Cullen, T.S. (1900). *Cancer of the Uterus*. (New York: Appleton)

36. Kurman, R.J., Kaminski, P.F. and Norris, H.J. (1985). The behavior of endometrial hyperplasia. A long term study of 'untreated' hyperplasia in 137 patients. *Cancer*, **56**, 403–12

37. Robboy, S.J. and Bradley, R. (1979). Changing trends and prognostic features in endometrial cancer associated with exogenous estrogen therapy. *Obstet. Gynecol.*, **54**, 269–77

38. Press, M.F. and Scully, R.E. (1985). Endometrial 'sarcomas' complicating ovarian thecoma, polycystic ovarian disease and estrogen therapy. *Gynecol. Oncol.*, **21**, 135–54

39. Gambrell, R.D. Jr. (1982). The menopause: benefits and risks of estrogen–progestogen replacement therapy. *Fertil. Steril.*, **37**, 457–74

40. Nachtigall, L.E., Nachtigall, R.H., Nachtigall, R.B. and Beckman, E.M. (1979). Estrogen replacement: a prospective study in the relationship to carcinoma and cardiovascular and metabolic problems. *Obstet. Gynecol.*, **54**, 74–9

41. Studd, J.W.W., Thom, M.H., Paterson, M.E.L. and Wade-Evans, T. (1980). The prevention and treatment of endometrial pathology in postmenopausal women receiving exogenous estrogens. In Pasetto, N., Paoletti, R. and Ambrus, J.L. (eds.) *The Menopause and Postmenopause*, pp. 127–39. (Lancaster, England: MTP Press)

42. Whitehead, M., Townsend, P.T., Pryse-Davies, J., Ryder, T.A. and King, R.J.B. (1981). Effects of estrogen and progestins on the biochemistry and morphology of the postmenopausal endometrium. *N. Engl. J. Med.*, **305**, 1599–605

43. Gambrell, R.D. Jr. (1986). The role of hormones in the etiology and prevention of endometrial cancer. *Clin. Obstet. Gynecol.*, **13**, 695–723

44. Gambrell, R.D. Jr. (1989). Use of progestogens in postmenopausal women. *Int. J. Fertil.*, **34**, 315–21

45. Campbell, S. and Whitehead, M. (1977). Oestrogen therapy and the menopausal syndrome. *Clin. Obstet. Gynecol.*, **4**, 31–48

46. Kistner, R.W. (1970). The effects of progestational agents on hyperplasia and carcinoma *in situ* of the endometrium. *Int. J. Obstet. Gynecol.*, **8**, 1563–79

47. Muechler, E.K., Bonfiglio, T., Choate, J. and Huang, K.E. (1986). Pregnancy induced with menotropins in a woman with polycystic ovaries, endometrial hyperplasia, and adenocarcinoma. *Fertil. Steril.*, **46**, 973–5

48. Kaufman, D.W., Shapiro, S.B., Slone, D., Rosenberg, L., Miettinen, O.S., Stolley, P.D., Knapp, R.C., Leavitt, T. Jr., Watring, W.G., Rosenhein, N.B., Lewis, J.L. Jr., Schottenfeld, D. and Engle, R.J. Jr. (1980). Decreased risk of endometrial cancer among oral contraceptive users. *N. Engl. J. Med.*, **303**, 1045–8

49. Weiss, N.S. and Sayetz, T.A. (1980). Incidence of endometrial cancer in relation to the use of oral contraceptives. *N. Engl. J. Med.*, **302**, 551–4

50. Hulka, B.S., Chambless, L.E., Kaufman, D.G., Fowler, W.C. Jr. and Greenberg, B.G. (1982). Protection against endometrial carcinoma by combination-product oral contraceptives. *J. Am. Med. Assoc.*, **247**, 475–7

51. Henderson, B.E., Casagrande, J.T., Pike, M.C., Mack, T., Rosario, I. and Duke, A. (1983). The epidemiology of endometrial cancer in young women. *Br. J. Cancer*, **47**, 749–56

Index